Besma HAMDI
Nouha Boubaker
Sabrine Louhaichi

COVID-19 pneumopathy

Besma HAMDI
Nouha Boubaker
Sabrine Louhaichi

COVID-19 pneumopathy

Predictors of poor prognosis

ScienciaScripts

Imprint

Cover image: www.ingimage.com

This book is a translation from the original published under ISBN 978-620-6-72352-3.

Publisher:
Sciencia Scripts
is a trademark of
Dodo Books Indian Ocean Ltd. and OmniScriptum S.R.L publishing group

120 High Road, East Finchley, London, N2 9ED, United Kingdom
Str. Armeneasca 28/1, office 1, Chisinau MD-2012, Republic of Moldova, Europe
Printed at: see last page
ISBN: 978-620-8-26788-9

TABLE OF CONTENTS

INTRODUCTION

Coronavirus 2019 (COVID-19) is an emerging disease caused by severe acute respiratory syndrome coronavirus 2 (SARS-CoV-2) [1]. It began in Wuhan, China, in December 2019 and rapidly spread to become a global pandemic in March 2020. More than 450 million cases of COVID-19 have been reported by the World Health Organisation since the start of the pandemic [2].

COVID-19 primarily affects the respiratory tract, with a broad spectrum of clinical expression. Although the majority of cases are mild, up to 20% of patients develop severe forms of the disease, including acute respiratory distress syndrome, multi-visceral failure and even death.

The course of the disease can be marked by a number of complications, not only respiratory but also thrombotic, cardiac, neurological, inflammatory and others [3,4].

These severe forms are explained by the tissue lesions induced directly by SARS-CoV-2 and by those induced by the host's inflammatory response. Indeed, SARS-CoV-2 leads to a prolonged and excessive inflammatory response corresponding to the cytokine storm that causes severe alveolar lesions [5].

In several countries, the peaks of the epidemic have generated a high demand for hospital beds, mainly in intensive care units, and a shortage of medical supplies, particularly personal protective equipment.

In Tunisia, up to 6.62% of patients with COVID-19 had been hospitalised by 25 April 2021, including 19% in intensive care units, with an overall mortality rate of around 3.5%[6].

As a result, early detection of patients at risk of worsening in the short term is of great importance, both for their early and appropriate management, and for better use of limited medical resources.

In this context, studies first conducted in China, and more recently in Europe and the United States, have sought to identify early factors in the poor outcome of patients with SARS-CoV-2 pneumonia, based on clinical, radiological and biological criteria. These factors differed according to the populations studied. [4,7-9]

The aim of our study was to investigate the epidemiological, clinical, biological and radiological characteristics of SARS-CoV-2 pneumonia in patients admitted to a respiratory department, and to identify factors predictive of an unfavourable short-term outcome.

METHODS

1. Type of study :

This is a retrospective, descriptive study including patients hospitalised in the Pneumology Department B of the Abderrahmane Mami Hospital for management of SARS-CoV-2 pneumonia between October 2020 and April 2021.

2. Study population :

2.1. Inclusion criteria :

All patients admitted to the Pneumology Department B of the Abderrahmane Mami Hospital for management of SARS-CoV-2 pneumonia confirmed by reverse transcription-polymerase chain reaction (RT-PCR) were included in this study.

2.2. The study did not include :

- Patients who did not require oxygen therapy during their hospital stay
- Patients transferred to the department after a stay in the intensive care unit

2.3. The study did not include :

- Patients with unstable respiratory or haemodynamic conditions on admission, requiring immediate transfer to the intensive care unit
- Patients readmitted to our department for secondary worsening after discharge.

3. Study methodology :

3.1. Data collection :

For each patient, we recorded epidemiological, clinical, radiological, therapeutic and evolutionary data.

The following parameters were collected:

3.1.1. Epidemiological parameters :

✓ Age

✓ Sex

✓ Habits: smoking

✓ Medical and surgical history

3.1.2. Clinical parameters :

✓ Functional respiratory and extra-respiratory signs: cough, dyspnoea, haemoptysis, chest pain, digestive signs (diarrhoea, vomiting), ear, nose and throat (ENT) signs (anosmia, agueusia, odynophagia), neurological signs ....

✓ General signs: fever, asthenia, anorexia, etc.

✓ Physical examination: weight, height, body mass index (BMI) (Appendix 1), temperature, respiratory rate (RR), peripheral oxygen saturation (SpO2), pulmonary auscultation, blood pressure, pulse.

We have also specified for our patients:

✓ The date of onset of symptoms

✓ The consultation period

✓ Treatment taken before hospitalisation (antibiotics, corticosteroids, etc.)

✓ Total length of hospital stay

3.1.3. Paraclinical parameters :

A- Biochemical and haematological analyses :

Biochemical and haematological tests included CBC, serum urea and creatinine, blood ionogram, blood glucose, liver function (transaminases, alkaline phosphatases, gamma glutamyl transpeptidase), C-reactive protein (CRP), creatine phosphokinase (CPK), lactate dehydrogenase (LDH), D-dimers. Anemia was defined as haemoglobin <12 g/dl, hyperleukocytosis as white blood cells $>10,000$ El/mm^3, neutrophilic polynucleosis as neutrophils (PNN) >7500/mm^3, lymphopenia as lymphocytes <1500 El/mm^3, thrombocytopenia as platelets $<150,000$/mm^3.The upper limits for CRP, aspartate aminotransferase(ASAT), alanine aminotransferase(ALAT) and CPK were set at : 20mg/L, 30IU/L, 35IU/L and 195IU/L respectively.

B- Microbiological samples :

All patients had a nasopharyngeal swab taken either before hospitalisation or on admission. The swab was sent for testing for SARS-CoV-2 by RT-PCR.

C- Thoracic imaging :

Most patients had undergone radiological investigation, at least by means of a thoracic CT scan.

The following data were noted:

-Type of parenchymal lesions: ground glass, condensation, crazy paving, etc.

-Degree of parenchymal involvement

-Presence of pleural and/or pericardial fluid effusion, pneumothorax or pneumomediastinum

With regard to parenchymal involvement, we used the visual scale recommended by the French Society of Radiology (SFR) and the European Society of Radiology to assess the extent of lesions [10], defining 5 categories: minimal involvement (10), moderate involvement (11-25%), significant involvement (26-50%), severe involvement (51-75%) and critical involvement (>75%).

Patients presenting signs of a complication underwent additional imaging: thoracic angioscan, brain scan, abdominal scan, ultrasound of the lower limbs....

3.1.4. Therapeutic management :

Therapeutic management was based on the recommendations of the French National Authority for Health Evaluation and Accreditation (INEAS) in the September 2020 version[11].

A-Oxygen therapy :

Oxygen therapy was provided by :

• Nasal cannula (LN) if oxygen flow <6 litres / minute

• High concentration mask (MHC) if oxygen flow 6 litres / minute

• High-flow nasal oxygen therapy (HFO) or non-invasive ventilation (NIV) if oxygen requirements exceed 15 litres.

B-Corticosteroid therapy :

Systemic corticosteroid therapy was prescribed for all patients.

Dexamethasone 6mg/day or hydrocortisone hemisuccinate 100mg x 2/d was used for up to 10 days.

C-Anticoagulation :

-All patients were placed on preventive anticoagulation according to weight and BMI.

► In patients with normal renal function :

• BMI < 30: enoxaparin 0.4 ml/d

• BMI 30: enoxaparin 0.4 ml x 2/d

• Weight > 120 kg: enoxaparin 0.6 ml x 2/d

► In the presence of renal insufficiency with creatinine clearance < 30 ml/mn :

• Heparin sodium 1-2 mg/kg/d or 100-200 IU/kg/d

• Or calciparin 5000 IU x 2/d

-Patients presenting a thromboembolic complication were put on curative anti-coagulation based on :

• Enoxaparin 100IU/Kg x 2/d, followed by anti-vitamin K (AVK) therapy

• Or unfractionated heparin if low molecular weight heparins (LMWH) are contraindicated.

3.1.5. Evolution :

We have defined :

• **A favourable outcome**: complete resolution or clinically significant improvement in all signs and symptoms of the disease with weaning from oxygen or discharge on home oxygen therapy in patients with chronic respiratory disease at the stage of chronic respiratory failure and in patients who had developed pulmonary fibrosis post COVID-19.

• **An unfavourable outcome**: death or transfer to an intensive care unit

-the main complications were :

• Respiratory: acute respiratory distress syndrome (ARDS), spontaneous barotrauma such as pneumothorax or pneumomediastinum.

• Thromboembolic: venous thrombosis, pulmonary embolism, arterial thrombosis, disseminated micro-emboli, ischaemic strokes

• Cardiovascular: myocarditis, rhythm disorders, heart failure, acute coronary syndrome

• Acute renal failure (defined according to the KDIGO 2012 guidelines as an increase in blood creatinine of 0.3mg/dl (26.5ymol/l) in 48 hours or an increase in blood creatinine of 0.3mg/dl (26.5ymol/l) in 48 hours or an increase in blood creatinine of 0.3mg/dl (26.5ymol/l) in 48 hours).1.5 baseline creatinine in seven days and/or diuresis<0.5ml/kg/h in six hours)

• Rhabdomyolysis (defined as a CPK level greater than 5 times normal)

• Cytolysis (defined as transaminase levels above 5 times normal)

4. Definitions of variables :

The clinical forms of SARS-CoV-2 pneumonia are defined according to the INEAS recommendations in appendix 2 :

✓ Asymptomatic form: RT-PCR positive with no clinical signs

✓ Minor form: No pneumonia, mild dry cough, malaise, headache, muscle pain, anosmia, agueusia, no dyspnoea

✓ Moderate form: Pneumonia without signs of severity (cough, mild dyspnoea, FR

< 30 cycles/minute, SpO2 94%)

✓ Severe form: Dyspnoea, FR30 cycles/minute and/or SpO2 < 94% on room air

✓ Critical form: Vital distress, shock, sepsis and/or organ failure and/or the need for invasive or non-invasive respiratory assistance.

Acute respiratory distress syndrome (ARDS) is defined according to the Berlin 2012 criteria in appendix 3 by[12] :

✓ Acute respiratory failure within 7 days of the initial attack (pulmonary or extra-pulmonary pathology)

✓ Bilateral pulmonary opacities on imaging

✓ Pulmonary oedema in which hydrostatic involvement is not predominant,

✓ Hypoxaemia defined by an arterial oxygen pressure (PaO2) / inspired oxygen fraction (FiO2) ratio 300 in a patient ventilated with a positive expiratory pressure (PEP) 5 cmH2O.

5. Statistical analysis :

The data were entered and coded using SPSS Version 21 software.

The data were processed statistically in two stages: the first descriptive and the second analytical.

5.1. Descriptive study :

• We calculated simple frequencies and relative frequencies (percentages) for the qualitative variables.

• We calculated means and standard deviations and determined the extreme values for the quantitative variables.

5.2. Analytical study :

• We conducted a univariate and multivariate analysis comparing all the data collected above in patients with a poor outcome and the rest of the patients in order to specify the prognostic factors of SARS-CoV-2 pneumopathy.

• **Comparison of means**: The Student's T test was used to compare the means of two independent samples. Means for non-dichotomous categorical variables were compared using the ANOVA test when their distribution was normal, and the non-parametric Kruskall-Wallis test in other cases.

• **Percentage comparisons**: Percentage comparisons were made using Pearson's chi-square test. If this test was not valid, the comparison was made using Fisher's two-tailed exact test.

• Risk factors were identified by calculating the odds ratio.

• To identify the risk factors independently linked to poor outcome, we performed a multivariate analysis using top-down binary logistic regression.

• In all statistical tests, the significance level was set at 0.05.

6. Ethical considerations :

We declare that there is no conflict of interest in this work. Ethical considerations were respected by ensuring the anonymity of patient records and security in storing, sending and receiving information.

7. Bibliographic research :

We used the following keywords COVID 19 - SARS-CoV-2 - Viral pneumonia - gravity - risk factor - evolution - prognosis.

The main search engines used were : Pubmed - Science direct - Google Scholar.

The references were entered and organised using ZOTERO software.

RESULTS

1. Descriptive study :

Over a 6-month period, 300 patients were selected. The overall distribution of patients is shown in the flow chart in Figure 1.

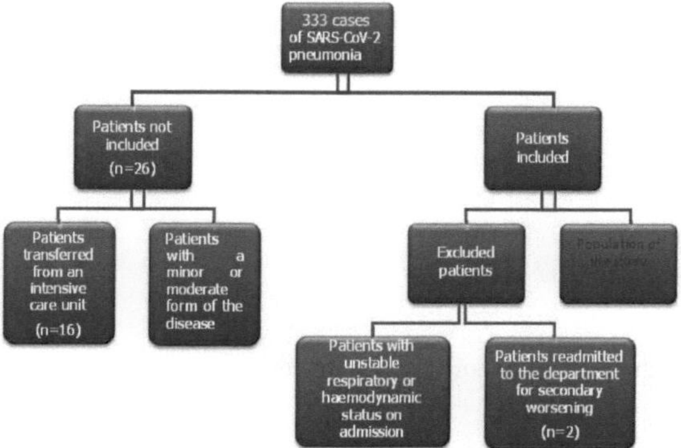

Figure 1: Overall distribution of patients

1.1. Epidemiological characteristics :

1.1.1. Age :

The median age of patients was 65, with extremes ranging from 18 to 91. The majority of patients were aged over 60 (n=200), representing 66.7% of cases (**Figure 2**).

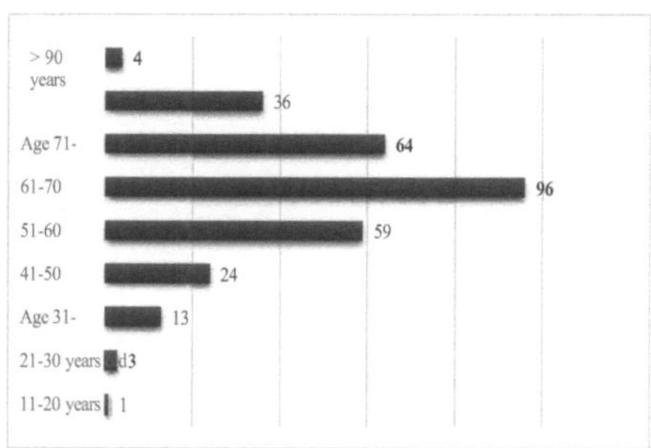

Figure 2: Breakdown of patients by age group

1.1.2. Gender :

Males predominated (n=174; 58%), with a sex ratio of 1.38.

1.1.3. Smoking :

Forty-four per cent of our patients were smokers (n=132). Of these patients, 43% had quit smoking before being admitted to our department. A study of smoking habits by sex showed that 91.7% of men and 8.3% of women smoked, with an average of 27 and 10 pack-years respectively (Figure 3).

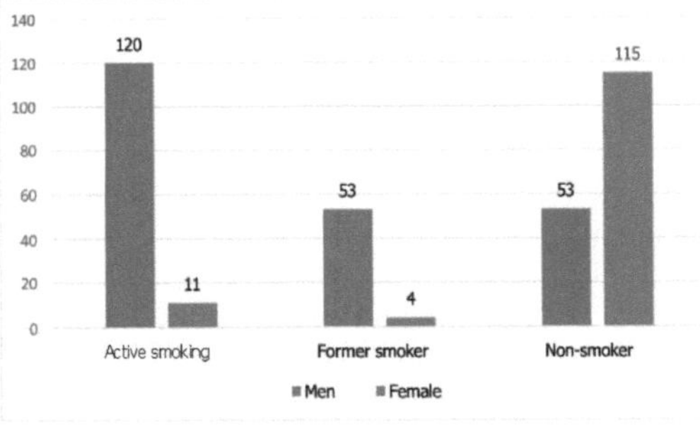

Figure 3: Breakdown of patients by sex and smoking status

1.1.4. Comorbidities :

The majority of our patients had at least one comorbidity (n=241; 80.3%). **Table I** illustrates the different comorbidities present in our patients. **Table I:** Prevalence of comorbidities

Medical conditions and medical history	Number of patients (n)	Percentage (%)
Cardiovascular diseases	**199**	**66,3**
HTA	136	45,3
Coronary artery disease	36	12
ACFA	18	6
CMD	9	3
Respiratory diseases	**101**	**33,6**
COPD	45	15
Asthma	19	6,3
Bronchopulmonary cancer	14	4,7
DDB	13	4,3
Pulmonary fibrosis	6	2
Tuberculosis	4	1,3
Endocrinopathies	**136**	**45**
Diabetes	118	39,3
Hypothyroidism	17	5,7
Chronic renal failure	**9**	**3**
Neurological pathologies	**13**	**4,3**
Psychiatric conditions	**9**	**3**

HTA: Hypertension; ACFA: Atrial fibrillation cardiac arrhythmia; CMD: Dilated cardiomyopathy; COPD: Chronic obstructive pulmonary disease; DDB: Bronchial dilatation.

1.2. Clinical data :

1.2.1. Medication taken prior to admission :

Prior to admission to our department, 38.7% of patients (n=116) had taken antibiotics. Azithromycin was the antibiotic most commonly used either alone or in combination with another antibiotic (n=84; 72.4%), followed by amoxicillin-clavulanic acid (n=23), 3rd generation cephalosporins (n=9), fluorquinolones (n=3), aminoglycosides (n=3) and macrolides (n=2). Eleven per cent of patients had taken oral corticosteroids prior to hospitalisation.

1.2.2. Time to onset of symptoms :

Almost all the symptoms appeared during the 2 weeks prior to hospitalisation (n=264), i.e. 88% of cases (**Figure 4**).

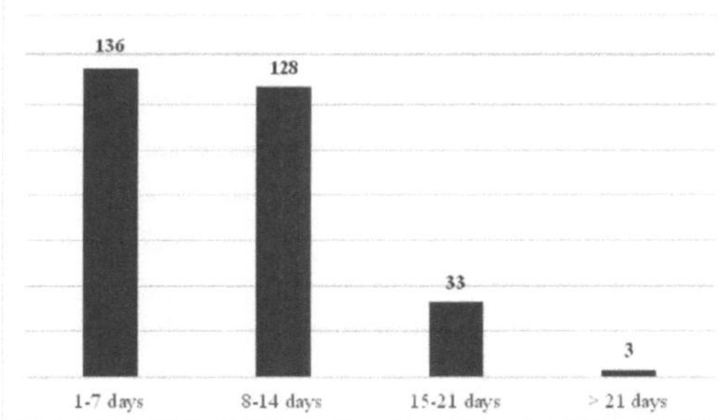

Figure 4: Distribution of patients by time to onset of symptoms

1.2.3. Functional signs :

Dyspnoea was the most frequent symptom (85.3%), followed by asthenia (78%), fever (72.3%) and cough (67.3%).

Table II shows the functional signs observed on patient admission.

Table II: Functional signs observed on admission

Functional signs	Number of patients (n)	Percentage (%)
General signs Asthenia	234	78
Fever	217	72,3
Myalgias	172	57,3
Anorexia	122	40,7
Headaches	118	39,3
Weight loss	22	7,3
Respiratory signs Dyspnoea	256	85,3
Cough	202	67,3
Chest pain	29	9,7
Haemoptysis	4	1,3
Digestive signs Diarrhoea	72	24
Vomiting	36	12
ENT signs Anosmia	34	11,3
Agueusia	32	10,7
Odynophagia	21	7
ENT: ear, nose and throat		

1.2.4. Physical examination :

1.2.4.1. Body Mass Index (BMI) :

BMI was calculated in 273 patients (91%). The mean BMI was 28.38±6.58 kg/m², with extremes ranging from 14 to 51 kg/m².The majority of patients had a BMI above the normal value (>24 kg/m2), i.e. 76% of cases (n=228), and 43% of them were obese (Figure 5). The distribution of patients by BMI is **shown in Figure 5**.

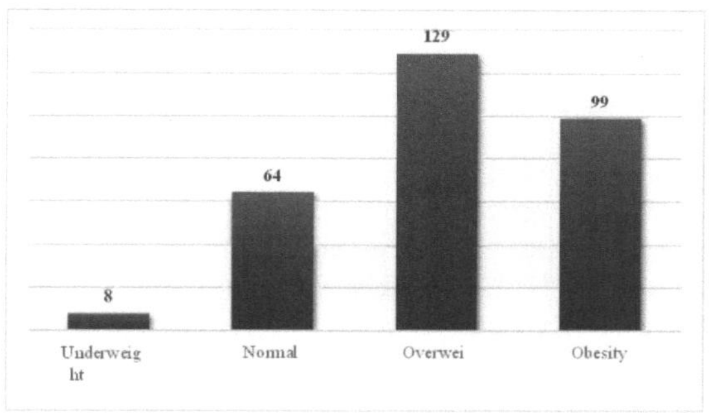

Figure 5: Breakdown of patients by BMI

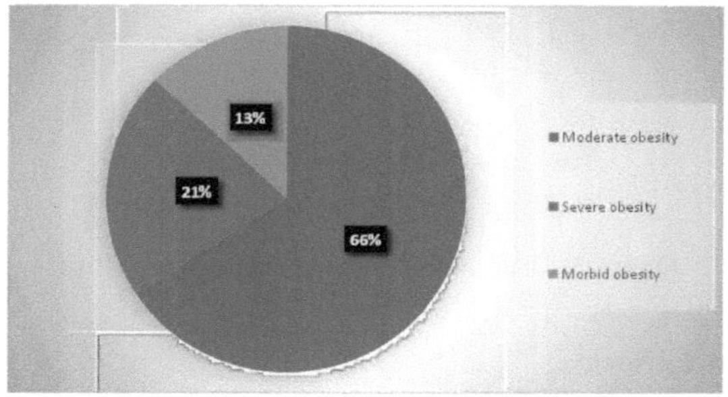

Figure 6: Distribution of patients according to degree of obesity

1.2.4.2. Vital parameters :

Polypnoea was the most frequent sign found on physical examination in half the patients, followed by tachycardia in 40 patients (13.3%) and fever in 32 patients (10.7%). The median oxygen flow rate required on admission was 6±6.2 L/min. It exceeded 15L/min in 17% of cases (n=51). (**Table** m) **Table III:** Patients' vital parameters

	Number of patients (n)	Percentage (%)
Fever	32	10,7
Tachycardia (HR>100 beats/minute)	40	13,3
Polypnoea (FR>18 cycles / minute)	150	50
O2 requirements		
<6 L/min	147	49
Between 6 and 15 L/min	102	34
15 L/min	51	17

HR: heart rate; RR: respiratory rate; O2: oxygen

1.3. Paraclinical data :

1.3.1. Biological check-up :

1.3.1.1. Blood count :

A complete blood count (CBC) study revealed hyperleukocytosis in 81 patients (27%), lymphopenia in 214 patients (71.3%), hyperbilirubinemia (11.3%), hyperbilirubinemia (11.3%) and hyperbilirubinemia (11.3%).thrombocytopenia in 37 patients (12.3%) and eosinopenia in 22 patients (7.3%) (**Figure 7**).

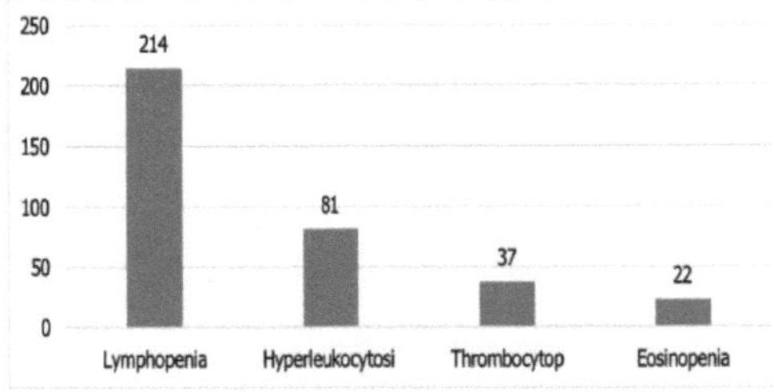

Figure 7: Distribution of blood count abnormalities

1.3.1.2. C-reactive protein :

The median level of C-reactive protein (CRP) was 112 milligrams/litre (mg/l) [2-455]. CRP 6 mg/l was observed in almost all patients (n=257), or 85.7% of cases.

1.3.1.3. Renal check-up :

Median creatinine and blood urea levels were 80 µmol/l [39-556] and 7 mmol/l [2-77] respectively. A total of 50 patients had renal failure (16.6%). Nine of these patients already had chronic renal failure, while the others had acute renal failure on admission (n=41, 13.6%).

1.3.1.4. Liver function tests :

Median ASAT and ALAT levels were 36 IU/l [11-530] and 29 IU/l [4-434] respectively. Hepatic cytolysis was observed in 55 patients (18.3%).

1.3.1.5. D-dimers :

The median D-dimer level was 720 µg/l [100-41750]. The majority of patients had high D-dimer levels (500µg/l) (n=195), i.e. 65% of cases.

1.3.1.6. Creatine phosphokinase :

The median CPK level was 85 IU/L, with extremes ranging from 8 to 4903 IU/L. Rhabdomyolysis was observed in 70 patients (23.3%).

1.3.1.7. Neutrophil to lymphocyte ratio (NLR) :

The mean NLR was 5.1 ±3.2 with extremes from 0.41 to 35.5. The NLR cut-off value of 4.9 was selected on the basis of a prognostic ROC curve study. The NLR was greater than 4.9 in 135 patients (45%).

Table IV shows the various biological results obtained on admission. Table IV: Biological profile of patients on admission.	observed in	our
Biological parameters Median	Interval	
Hb (g/dl) 13	[8-17]	
Granulocytes (El/mm3) 7800	[770-64000]	
Neutrophils (El/mm³) 5710	[580-30240]	
Lymphocytes (El/mm³) 1100	[300-14280]	
Eosinophils (El/mm³) 80	[0-800]	
Platelets (El/mm3) 236000	[11-662000]	
NLR 5,1	[0,41-35,3]	
PLR 228	[28-727]	
Urea (mmol/l) 7	[2-77]	
Creatinine (µmol/l) 80	[39-556]	
AST (IU/l) 36	[11-530]	
ALAT(IU/l) 29	[4-534]	
D-dimer (µg/l) 720	[100-41750]	
CRP (mg/l) 112	[2-455]	
LDH (IU/l) 366	[23-1504]	
CPK (IU/l) 108,5	[14-4738]	

HB: Haemoglobin; NLR: Neutrophil to lymphocyte ratio; PLR: Platelet to lymphocyte ratio; ASAT: Aspartate aminotransferase; ALAT: Alanine aminotransferase; CRP: C-reactive protein; LDH: Lactate dehydrogenase; CPK: Creatine phosphokinase.

1.3.2. Thoracic imaging :

Chest CT scans were performed in most patients (n=285; 95%). The majority of patients had more than 50% lung parenchyma involvement (n=164, 57.6%) (**Figure 8) (Appendices 4-5-6**).

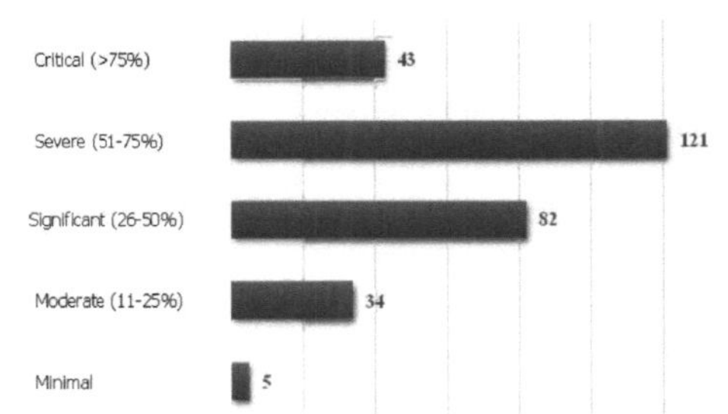

Figure 8: Distribution of patients according to degree of parenchymal involvement on chest CT scan

The majority of lesions were bilateral (n=279; 97.9%). Ground-glass lesions and condensations were observed in 95.8% and 67% of cases respectively (**Figure 9**).

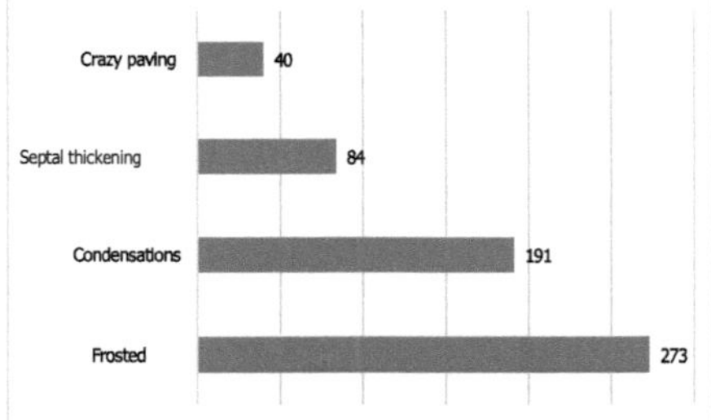

Figure 9: Breakdown of patients by type of lesion observed on chest CT scan

1.4. Therapeutic management :

1.4.1. Oxygen therapy :

All patients received oxygen therapy. The median oxygen flow rate on admission was 6 L/min, with extremes ranging from 1 to 60 L/min.

Figure 7 illustrates the oxygen therapy modalities.

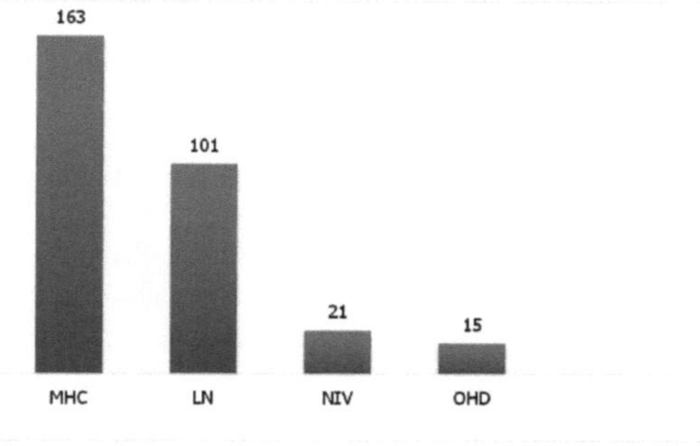

Figure 10: Oxygen therapy methods

1.4.2. Drug treatment :

1.4.2.1. Anticoagulants :

The majority of patients had taken anticoagulants as a preventive measure (n=212; 71%). The remainder of patients had received curative anticoagulation (n=88; 29%). Twenty patients were put back on anticoagulants as a preventive measure after pulmonary embolism had been ruled out.

Table V illustrates the different indications for curative anticoagulation.

Table V: Indications for curative anticoagulation

Indications for curative anticoagulation	**Number of patients (n)**		**Percentage (%)**	
Strong suspicion of pulmonary embolism	33		11	
Atrial fibrillation	26		8,6	
Confirmed pulmonary embolism	22		7,3	
Acute limb ischaemia inferior	4		1,3	
Multiple arterial thrombosis	2		0,6	
Deep vein thrombosis	1		0,3	
1.4.2.2. Corticosteroid therapy :				
All patients received dexamethasone-based corticosteroid therapy.	à	the dose	6mg/day	has been

The average duration of treatment was 8 days [1-10] but did not exceed 10 days.

1.4.2.3. Antibiotic therapy :

One or more antibiotics were administered in 27 patients (9%). Ceftriaxone and azithromycin were the 2 most commonly used drugs in patients treated with antibiotics, accounting for 37.2% and 25.6% of cases respectively.

Table VI below illustrates the indications for antibiotic therapy.

Table VI: Indications for antibiotic therapy

Indications for antibiotic therapy	Number of patients (n)	Percentage (%)
Superinfection of DDB	3	1
PBC superinfection	3	1
Abscessed pneumonia	1	0,3
Bronchial superinfection in COPD	20	6,6
DDB: bronchial dilatation; CBP: cancer	bronchopulmonary; COPD :	Bronchopneumopathy chronic obstructive

1.5. Evolution :

1.5.1. Positive trends :

Two-thirds of patients had a favourable outcome (n=200; 67%). Eleven patients required home oxygen therapy. The indications for home oxygen therapy are presented in **Table VII**.

Table VII: Indications for home oxygen therapy

Indications for home oxygen therapy	Number of patients (n)	Percentage (%)
Chronic respiratory disease at CKD stage Pulmonary fibrosis	10 5	3,3 1,6
DDB	3	1
COPD	2	0,6
Post COVID-19 pulmonary fibrosis	1	0,3

CRI: chronic respiratory failure; bronchial dilatation; COPD: chronic obstructive pulmonary disease.

Curative anticoagulation for 6 months was prescribed for patients who developed thromboembolic complications during hospitalisation (n=17). Preventive anticoagulation was prescribed for the remaining patients (n=183) for an average of 15 days, including the period of hospitalisation.

1.5.2. Unfavourable trend :

1.5.2.1. Transfer to the intensive care unit :

During their hospitalisation, 84 patients were transferred to the intensive care unit for ARDS (28%). The median age of patients transferred was 63 ±10 years. The time to transfer to the intensive care unit after admission was 10±7 days.

1.5.2.2. Deaths :

Death occurred in 16 patients (5%) with a mean survival time of 7 ± 4 days. The median age of patients who died was 79 ±10 years. The leading cause of death was ARDS (n=13), followed by acute cardiogenic pulmonary oedema (n=3). Figure 11 shows the distribution of patients according to clinical course.

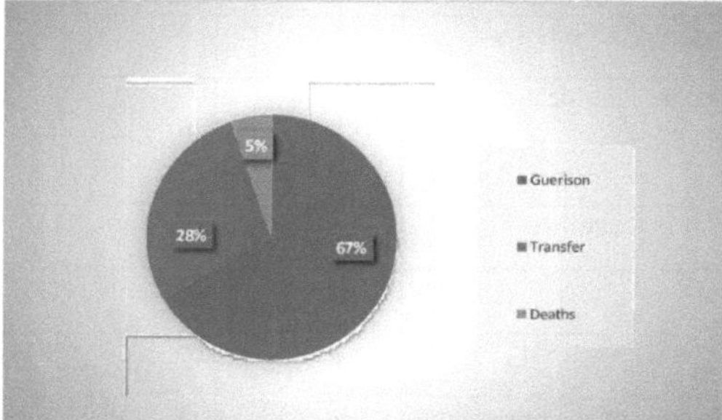

Figure 11: Breakdown of patients by clinical course

1.5.3. Complications :

One or more complications occurred in 217 patients during their treatment (72%). The most frequent complication was ARDS observed in 97 patients (32%) followed by acute renal failure in 41 patients (13.6%) and pulmonary embolism in 22 patients (7.3%). **(Table VIII)**

Table IX: Breakdown of patients admitted to hospital Frequency (n)	acco rdin g to	the type	fro m	complications during Percentage(%)
Pulmonary complications ARDS		97		32
Pneumothorax		3		1
Pneumo mediastinum		2		0,6
Thromboembolic complications Pulmonary embolism		22		7,3
Deep vein thrombosis		1		0,3
Multiple arterial thrombosis		2		0,6
Cardiovascular complications ACFA		8		2,6
Suspicion of myocarditis		4		1,3
Pericarditis		3		1
BAV		2		0,6
Acute ischaemia of the lower limbs		4		1,3
Bradycardia		5		1,6
OAP		10		3,3
Acute renal failure		41		13,6
Neurological complications				
Hallucinations		3		1
Agitation		10		3,3

ARDS: Acute respiratory distress syndrome; AFCA: Atrial fibrillation cardiac arrhythmia; AVB: Atrioventricular block; APO: Acute pulmonary oedema.

1.6. Length of hospital stay :

The average length of hospital stay for patients was 9.5 ±6 days. **(Table IX).**

Table X: Average length of hospital stay for patients

	Average (days)	Standard deviation
Recovered (n=200)	9,9	5,9
Deceased (n=16)	7	4,6
Transferred (n=84)	10	7
Total (n=300)	9,5	6

2. Analytical study :

2.1. Univariate study :

2.1.1. General characteristics :

In our study, there was no significant association between pre-admission drug intake, comorbidities and poor patient outcomes. In addition, unfavourable clinical outcomes were more common in men (OR=1.95; 95% CI:1.34-2.85; p<0.001) (**Table X**).

Table XI : Variation of evolution according to the characteristics and co-morbidities.

General characteristics

Favourable outcome (n=200)

Unfavourable trend p (n=100)

Age65 years		104(52%)	56(56%)0,51	
Men		101 (50,5%)	73 (73%)	
Gender		< 0,001		
	Woman	99 (49,5%)	27 (27%)	
Tobacco		81 (40,5%)	51 (51%)	0,084
	Assets	45(22,5%)	30(30%)	0,09
	Weaned	36(18%)	21(21%)	0,56
Antibiotic therapy before admission		84(42%)	32(32%)	0,09
Corticosteroid therapy before admission		25(12,5)	8(8%)	0,16
Comorbidities		158 (79%)	83 (83%)	0,411
Diabetes		79 (39,5%)	39 (39%)	0,933
HTA		86 (43%)	50 (50%)	0,251
Coronary artery disease		24 (12%)	12 (12%)	1
CMD		4 (2%)	5 (5%)	0,166
ACFA		11 (5,5%)	7 (7%)	0,606
Renal insufficiency		5 (2,5%)	4 (4%)	0,487
COPD		26 (13%)	19 (19%)	0,170
Asthma		14 (7%)	5 (5%)	0,503
Bronchopulmonary cancer		8 (4%)	6 (6%)	0,562
DDB		10 (5%)	3 (3%)	0,555
Pulmonary fibrosis		5(2,5%)	1(1%)	0,7
Pulmonary tuberculosis		3 (1,5%)	1 (1%)	1
Neuropathies		9 (4,5%)	4 (4%)	0,8
Hypothyroidism		13 (6,5%)	4 (4%)	0,377
Psychiatric conditions		7 (3,5%)	2 (2%)	0,723

HTA: Hypertension; ACFA: Atrial fibrillation cardiac arrhythmia; CMD: Dilated cardiomyopathy; COPD: Chronic obstructive pulmonary disease; DDB: Bronchial dilatation.

2.1.2. Clinical parameters :

2.1.2.1. Functional signs :

There were no significant differences between the symptoms reported in the two groups, with the exception of diarrhoea, which was associated with a poor prognosis (OR=1.78; 95% CI:1.1-2.89; p=0.01).

Table XI illustrates the relationship between functional signs and patient outcome.

Table XII: Variation in progression according to functional signs

Functional signs	Favourable evolution (n=200)	Unfavourable trend (n=100)	p
Time to onset of symptoms (days)	9 [1-34]	7 [3-25]	0,054
Myalgia	116 (58%)	56 (56%)	0,741
Headaches	86 (43%)	32 (32%)	0,066
Dyspnoea	168 (84%)	88 (88%)	0,356
Cough	135(67,5%)	67 (67%)	0,931
Chest pain	20 (10%)	9 (9%)	0,782
Haemoptysis	1 (0,5%)	3 (3%)	0,110
Diarrhoea	57 (28,5%)	15 (15%)	0,010
Vomiting	28 (14%)	8 (8%)	0,132
Anosmia	22 (11%)	12 (12%)	0,797
Agueusia	18 (9%)	14 (14%)	0,186
Odynophagia	11 (5,5%)	10 (10%)	0,150
Anorexia	83 (41,5%)	39 (39%)	0,678
Asthenia	162 (81%)	72 (72%)	0,076
Weight loss	16 (8%)	6 (6%)	0,531

2.1.2.2. Physical signs :

Patients in the second group had a higher BMI (p=0.036). Adverse outcomes were more common in patients with polypnoea (p<0.001) and those requiring high oxygen flow on admission (OR=4.8; 95% CI:2.8- 8.3; p<0.001).

Table XIII: Changes in vital parameters

Evolution Physical signs favourable	Unfavourable trend	p
(n=200)	(n=100)	
Temperature (°C)37 [36-40]	37 [36-39]	0,535
Fever 135(67,5%)	82 (82%)	0,08
BMI (Kg/m2)27 [14-45]	28 [17-45]	0,036
Overweight 88(44%)	36(36%)	0,2
Moderate obesity42(21%)	23(23%)	0,297
Severe obesity 15(7,5%)	6(6%)	0,08
Morbid obesity 5(2,5%)	8(8%)	0,02
Need for Oxygen at5[1-30] (Litres/minute)	10[2-60]	< 0,001
Pouls85 [52-130]	87 [48-124]	0,876
Tachycardia27 (13.5%)	13 (13%)	0,904
FR (Cycles/minute) 20 [12-47]	22 [12-40]	< 0,001

BMI: Body Mass Index; RR: Respiratory Rate

2.1.3. Variation in patient outcome according to biological parameters :

Biological parameters on admission associated with clinical deterioration were hyperleukocytosis (p=0.006), thrombocytopenia (p=0.013), elevated C-reactive protein (p=0.001), elevated blood creatinine (p=0.007), elevated neutrophil/lymphocyte ratio (p=0.001), elevated D-dimer (p=0.01) and rhabdomyolysis (p<0.001). Tables XIV and XIV summarise the results of the univariate study looking for biological factors associated with poor outcome. The distribution of rates for the various biological parameters is shown in **Figures 11-17.**

Table XV: Variation in progression according to biological results

Favourable evolution Biological check-up (n=200)		Unfavourable trend (n=100)	p
Haemoglobin (g/dl)	13 [9-17]	12 [8-16]	0,479
Haemoglobin<12g/dl	92 (46%)	49 (49%)	0,624
Leukocytes (103 El/mm3)	7,2 [3-64]	8,55 [0,77-22,1]	0,456
Leukocytes10000 El/mm3	44 (22%)	37 (37%)	0,006
Lymphocytes<1500 El/mm3	136(68%)	78(78%)	0,056
PNE<40 El/mm3	16(8%)	6(6%)	0,6
NLR (average)	5,3	7,4	0,001
Platelets (103 El/mm3)	240 [0,11-662]	212 [10,6-623]	0,028
Platelets<150000 El/mm3	18 (9%)	19 (19%)	0,013
PLR(average)	228,4	228,7	0,9
Blood creatinine (µmol/l)	84±41	105±67	0,007
Hepatic cytolysis	33 (16,5%)	22 (22%)	0,246
CRP (mg/l)	112 ±76	157,8 ±91	<0,001
D-dimer (µg/l)	1759±3636	1928±3887	0,010
CPK (IU/l)	92 [14-3099]	132 [16-4738]	0,035
Rhabdomyolysis34	(17%)	36 (36%)	< 0,001

PNE: polynuclear cellseosinophils;
NLR:neutrophil/lymphocyte ratio; PLR: platelet to lymphocyteratio; CRP: C-reactive protei; CPK: creatine phosphokinase

Table XVI: Biological risk factors for aggravation

	OR	95% CI
Hyperleukocytosis	2,08	[1,23-3,52]
Thrombocytopenia	2,37	[1,18-4,75]
High NLR	2,1	[1,1-3,16]
Elevated CRP	11,3	[11,2-67]
Rhabdomyolysis	2,74	[1,58-4,76]
High D-dimer levels	2	[1,17-3,41]

NLR: neutrophil/lymphocyte ratio; CRP: C-reactive protein

2.1.4. Variation in evolution according to lesions tomodensitométriques

The severity of lung damage on CT and septal thickening were risk factors for worsening (p 0.001 and 0.05 respectively) (**Table XV**).

Table XVII: Radiological aggravation risk factors

	Evolution favourable	Evolution unfavourable	P
	(n=200)	(n=100)	
Severe disease (>50%)	101(50%)	63(63%)	0,001
Frosted glass	188(94%)	85(85%)	0,3
Septal thickening	48(24%)	36(36%)	0,05
Crazy paving	25(13%)	15(15%)	0,06
Condensations	134(67%)	57(57%)	0,3
Pulmonary embolism	15(7,5%)	6(6%)	0,8

2.2. Multivariate study :

The multivariate study identified the following independent risk factors for poor outcome:

- The male sex

- Oxygen requirements on admission

- A high neutrophil/lymphocyte ratio

Factors predictive of poor outcome in patients hospitalised with SARS-CoV-2 pneumonia are detailed in **Table XVI.**

Table XVIII: Independent factors of poor evolution

	P	OR	95% CI
Male sex	<0,001	4,5	2,04-10,1
Oxygen requirements on admission	<0,001	2,3	2,1-3,4
NLR	0,01	1,8	1,09-3,04

NLR: neutrophil/lymphocyte ratio

• After ROC curve analysis, the optimal threshold for oxygen requirements on admission was found to be 5.5 litres, with a sensitivity of 75% and a specificity of 61%, an area under the curve equal to 0.75 and a p<0.001. (**Figure 12**)

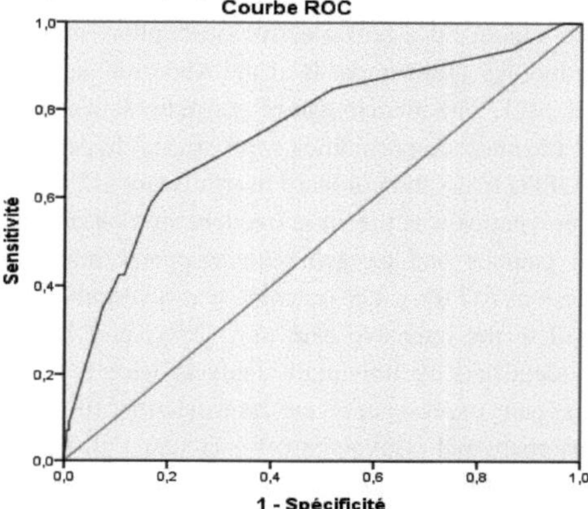

Figure 12: ROC curve of the optimal threshold of oxygen requirements on admission

DISCUSSION

In order to identify the poor prognostic factors of SARS-CoV-2 pneumopathy in a pneumology setting, we conducted a retrospective descriptive study including 300 patients hospitalised in the Pneumology Department B of the Abderrahmane Mami Hospital between October 2020 and April 2021. The median age of our patients was 65 ± 13 years, with a sex ratio of 1.38. The most common comorbidities were arterial hypertension (45.3%), followed by diabetes (39.3%), COPD (15%) and coronary heart disease (12%). Dyspnoea was the main symptom (85.3%) and polypnoea was the most frequent sign on physical examination (50%). On admission, 51% of patients had oxygen requirements6L/min and more than half had extensive radiological lesions (57.6%). The outcome was favourable in 200 patients (67%), 84 patients were transferred to the intensive care unit (28%) and 16 patients died (6%). The prognostic factors we identified by univariate analysis were male sex ($p<10^{-3}$), digestive signs(p=0.01), high oxygen requirements on admission($p<10^{-3}$), higher BMI (p=0.03), polypnoea($p<10^{-3}$), parenchymal involvement greater than 50%(p=0.001), septal thickening(p=0.005) and several biological factors. The biological parameters on admission associated with a poor prognosis were hyperleukocytosis (p=0.006), thrombocytopenia (p=0.013), elevated C-reactive protein (p=0.001), elevated blood creatinine (p=0.007), elevated neutrophil to lymphocyte ratio (p=0.001), elevated d-dimer (p=0.01) and rhabdomyolysis ($p < 0.001$). The analytical study looking for independent predictive factors of poor outcome identified male sex as a risk factor (OR=4.5; 95% CI :2.07-10.1; $p<10^{-3}$), oxygen requirements on admission5.5 litres (OR=2.3; 95% CI :2.1-3.4; $p<10^{-3}$) and a neutrophil to lymphocyte ratio4.9 (OR=1.8; 95% CI :1.09-3.04; p=0.01).

Highlights:

• The relevance of the subject study us a allowed to study the characteristics of patients hospitalised in a pneumology department for SARS-CoV-2 pneumopathy and to identify the prognostic factors for this pathology using a multivariate analysis.

• Large sample size: To our knowledge, this study is the largest Tunisian series reported on the prognostic factors of SARS-CoV-2 pneumonia.

Weaknesses :

• The retrospective and monocentric nature of our study.
• Some clinical and/or biological data missing from the files.
• There was no comparison with a group that had a minor or moderate form of SARS-CoV-2 pneumonia.

In December 2019, the appearance of several cases of pneumonia of unknown origin in Wuhan, Hubei province in China led to the identification, in January 2020, of a new coronavirus, called severe acute respiratory syndrome coronavirus 2 (SARS-CoV-2) by the Coronavirus Working Group of the International Committee on Taxonomy of Viruses [13]. Human-to-human transmission led to the rapid spread of the virus, first throughout China and then throughout the world, causing a pandemic [2]. The disease shook the world because of the speed with which it spread, its high lethality and its socio-economic impact.

In Tunisia, the first wave of the COVID-19 pandemic began on 2 March 2020. A number of health measures were rapidly implemented, ranging from border closures to a general health lockdown. These measures helped to slow the spread of the pandemic. The total number of confirmed COVID-19 cases up to 08 April 2020 was 643 [14], leading to the gradual lifting of health measures and the reopening of borders on 27 June 2020. With the start of the second wave, the country saw an exponential increase in the number of cases declared COVID19 positive. This time, more severe forms of the disease were observed, with a shortage of hospital beds, especially in intensive care units. In June 2021, the occupancy rate of hospital beds reached 100% in many governorates [15].

It was therefore necessary for clinicians to recognise the risk factors for the unfavourable evolution of SARS-CoV-2 pneumonia in order to identify patients at risk of complications and optimise the management of resources and supply. capacity, particularly in intensive care. The aim of this study was to provide a descriptive overview of SARS-CoV-2 pneumonia and to identify prognostic factors. The median age of our patients was 65 years [18-91], comparable to that reported in the literature[16]. Advanced age has been identified as an independent predictor of mortality in SARS and MERS, two viruses that belong to the same coronavirus family[17]. This has also been demonstrated for SARS-CoV-2. In a cohort study of 66 million people, the risk of hospitalisation for COVID19 was 5 times higher and the risk of death was 100 times higher in people aged 85 and over compared with those aged 40-44[18]. In our study, advanced age was not associated with poor disease progression. This could be explained by the small size of our population. In line with our study, male predominance has been found in various international series [8,19,20].Lifestyle and behavioural differences between the sexes appear to be an important factor in explaining this male predominance. On the one hand, women have a lower prevalence of smoking and cardiovascular disease, which are associated with a poorer prognosis in patients with COVID-19. On the other hand, anxiety disorders are predominant in women, which could lead to more restrictive activities and social distancing in women [25].

Studies have sought to explain the effect of sex difference on disease prognosis by a higher expression of angiotensin-converting enzyme type 2 (ACE2) receptor in men [21,22]. Other studies have looked at the role of androgens and oestrogens in the severity and prognosis of the disease. Entry of SARS-CoV-2 into lung cells requires cleavage of the Spike protein by transmembrane serine protease 2 (TMPRSS2), a cellular protease whose expression is stimulated by androgens. This could explain the importance of mild forms in children with low expression of androgen receptors, as well as in patients being treated for prostate cancer and receiving anti-androgens[22,23]. Furthermore, experimental studies in animals suggest that oestrogens lower the expression of ACE2 in the cell membrane and inhibit the interaction of SARS-CoV-2 with ACE2 in the lungs[24]. This protective effect of oestrogen could explain the high incidence of infection and the severe forms of the disease in post-menopausal women. Indeed, a multicentre Chinese study conducted by Ding et al showed that the menopause is an independent risk factor for the severity of COVID19, while estradiol (E2) and antimüllerian hormone (AMH) are negatively correlated with the severity of the disease[25]. Another study including 459 patients showed no significant association between sex and mortality in patients aged over 65, in contrast to younger patients, suggesting a protective role for oestrogens[26].In line with the literature, the results of our multivariate analysis show that male gender is a factor in poor prognosis.

The prevalence of smoking was much higher in our patients than in the literature[27]. This could be explained by the high frequency of smoking in Tunisia[28].

As for its prognostic value, numerous studies have investigated the relationship between smoking and the prognosis of SARS-CoV-2 pneumonia, with controversial results. Indeed, some authors have reported that patients who smoke have a poor clinical outcome. A meta-analysis including 32849 patients hospitalised for COVID-19 showed that active smokers had an increased risk of severe disease (RR=1.8), disease progression (RR=2.18), need for mechanical ventilation (RR=1.2) and in-hospital mortality (RR=1.26)[31].

In other studies such as ours, there was no significant association between smoking and poor prognosis [32,33]. Thomas et al explained these results by the lack of detailed data on smoking status, the time between smoking cessation and the disease and a lack of adjustment for sex, age and smoking-related pathologies in certain studies [34].

One of the hypotheses put forward by certain authors is the protective effect of nicotine. However, prospective studies are needed to assess this hypothesis[35,36].
All the studies described that the presence of frequent comorbidities also increased the risk of worsening and death in patients with COVID-19 [37,38]. In our study, comorbidities were present in 80.3% of patients with patients. Hypertension was the most common comorbidity (45.3%), followed by diabetes (39.3%), coronary heart disease (12%) and COPD (15%).

A meta-analysis including 6,560 patients concluded that hypertension was associated with high mortality, increased use of intensive care and progression to acute respiratory distress syndrome[39]. This was explained by the fact that the virus enters host cells via its association with ACE2, which is involved in the renin-angiotensin-aldosterone system (RAAS). This system is thought to be spontaneously over-activated in hypertensive patients[40-42]. The COVID- 19 and hypertension (COVHYP) study in France and the BRACE-CORONA study in Brazil showed no association between prior treatment with ACE inhibitors and angiotensin II AT1 receptor antagonists (AIIRA) and poor patient prognosis[43,44]. These results concurred with those of the majority of published studies in favour of the absence of a deleterious effect of these drugs in patients with COVID-19[45].

Similarly, the protective effect of ACE inhibitors/ARA2 on severe forms of COVID-19 has not been demonstrated, despite the existence of experimental arguments in favour of this effect[46,47]. As in the case of hypertension, diabetes is a factor in unfavourable progression. This could be attributed to impaired innate immunity, chronic inflammation and elevated coagulation activity in these patients [48].

Indeed, its association with disease severity was reported by Matsushita et al in a meta-analysis of 51,845 patients. The results were similar in meta-analyses carried out in China and Italy [16,49,50].

In the French multicentre CORONADO study, the mortality rate was 11%, confirming the seriousness of COVID-19 in hospitalised diabetic patients. However, this rate was much lower in subjects with type 1 diabetes than in those with type 2 (5.4% versus 10.6%), in relation to a younger age [51]. Contrary to the studies cited above, our work did not show any association between these two comorbidities and the poor outcome of our patients. This could be explained on the one hand by the small size of our population compared with the series reported in the literature and on the other hand by the presence of unreported comorbidities such as neurodegenerative diseases, which are very common in these patients and which would probably be an independent factor in the poor outcome[52]. Our results could also be explained by the fact that the statistical analysis of our work did not take into account the stage of these comorbidities and the presence or absence of chronic complications such as diabetic neuropathy and hypertensive nephropathy.

Fifteen per cent of our patients had COPD. This incidence was higher than those reported in the literature. In a meta-analysis of 15 studies involving 2473 patients, the incidence of COPD was 2%. This could be explained by the lower incidence of smoking (9% versus 56% in our study)[53].

In addition, its association with poor outcome was well established in several studies. Indeed, in a multicentre study conducted in China, COPD was more frequent in patients with critical forms of COVID19 than in those with moderate forms of the disease (15.7% versus 2.5%; $p<0.001$)[54]. Similar results were reported by Javanmardi and Alqahtani with higher rates of intensive care unit hospitalisation and death in COPD patients[53,55].

Leung et al sought to explain this association by the greater expression of ACE2 in patients with COPD. However, the increased expression of ACE-2 in patients with COPD would not be sufficient in itself to explain the severity of the disease in these patients[56]. The comorbidities associated with COPD are also thought to be a factor in the worsening of the disease[53].

Contrary to the studies cited above, our work did not show any association between COPD and the poor outcome of our patients.

The prevalence of asthma was low in most studies [57-59]. This prevalence depended on the type of asthma. Patients with allergic asthma had a much lower risk of infection. This has been explained by several mechanisms, namely the excessive production of interleukin-4, interleukin-5, interleukin-13, specific immunoglobulin E (IgE) and eosinophils in atopic asthma. It has also been shown that ACE2 expression is lower in the nasal and bronchial epithelial cells of allergic individuals[59]. This is associated with excessive IL-13 production and regular use of inhaled corticosteroids[60,61].

Non-allergic asthma is associated with a higher risk of infection and poor prognosis. This is due to the higher expression of ACE-2, the older age of patients and the presence of co-morbidities such as obesity, diabetes and arterial hypertension [59].

As for the prognostic value of asthma, it has been established that it is not associated with poor disease progression. Indeed, the English study by Williamson et al, carried out on a population of more than 17 million patients, showed that asthma is not a poor prognostic factor, except in the case of very severe patients who had received oral systemic corticosteroids shortly before the infection [62].With regard to background treatment, it has been shown that inhaled corticosteroids or anti-IL5 or anti-IgE biotherapies have no impact on the frequency and severity of SARS-CoV-2 infection, unlike systemic corticosteroids, which have been correlated with disease severity [63,64]. In the present study, and in line with the literature, asthma was not associated with poor disease progression.In the clinical presentation of our patients, dyspnoea was the most frequent symptom (85.3%), followed by asthenia (78%), fever (72.3%) and cough (67.3%). These data are similar in other worldwide series [65,66].

As in our work, several studies have noted the importance of digestive signs in SARS-CoV-2 pneumonia. In the series by Pan et al, digestive manifestations accounted for 50.5% of all symptoms [19] . In another retrospective Chinese series of 1141 confirmed cases of COVID-19, 16
% of patients had isolated digestive symptoms[67]. SARS-CoV-2 has an affinity for the ACE2 receptor on human cells, which it uses to bind to and enter the cell. The ACE2 receptor is present in lung alveolar type 2 cells, but is also highly expressed in the digestive tract, suggesting that the virus can invade the enterocytes of the digestive tract [68,69]. However, digestive symptoms may be caused directly by viral invasion or may be secondary to lesions induced by the immune response [70,71].

In our study, only diarrhoea was associated with a poor prognosis. The same finding was reported by Jin et al in a retrospective study of 651 patients [20], which could be explained by the ionic disorders caused by diarrhoea. With regard to physical examination findings, obesity was found in 33% of our patients. Its prognostic role has been reported by several authors. In a meta-analysis including 4,444 participants, Jun Yang concluded that obese patients with COVID19 had more severe forms of the disease and a poorer prognosis than non-obese patients[72]. Comparable results were found in the United States and France[73-75]. Obesity has also been shown to increase the risk of intubation in intensive care units and the risk of death [76,77].

The pathophysiological mechanisms that may explain the association between obesity and severe forms of COVID-19 are : altered ventilatory mechanics, overexpression of ACE2 receptors, obesity-related hypercoagulability and excessive secretion of proinflammatory adipokines such as interleukin-6 (IL-6) and tumour necrosis factor alpha (TNFa), and comorbidities frequently associated with obesity such as arterial hypertension, diabetes and obstructive sleep apnoea syndrome[78].

In our study, although patients with a higher BMI had a worse prognosis, only morbid obesity was significantly associated with a poor prognosis. This could be explained by the fact that the majority of obese patients were younger (62±13 years versus 66±14 years; p=0.01).

Hypoxia requiring high oxygen flow was a frequent finding on physical examination in our population and was associated with poor disease progression. Our results were consistent with those in the literature. Indeed, in a systematic review of the literature by Izcovich including 207 studies and 75607 patients with COVID19, hypoxia increased the risk of progression of the disease to a severe form and of death (relative risk 4.69 and 5.40 respectively)[79].

Although all our patients were hypoxic, only half of them had polypnoea on admission. This was explained by the phenomenon of silent hypoxaemia observed in COVID-19, the pathophysiological mechanisms of which involve the conjunction of peripheral mechanisms dominated by the intra pulmonary shunt, the inadequacy of the ventilation/perfusion ratio, the loss of regulation of pulmonary perfusion and the presence of intravascular microthrombi and central mechanisms [80,81].

Also, the direct local action of the virus and the associated inflammatory reaction could disrupt the function of peripheral mechanoreceptors and chemoreceptors and thus contribute to silent hypoxaemia[80]. As a result, Gattioni et al suggested the existence of two major phenotypes of SARS-CoV-2 pneumonia: the type L phenotype and the type H phenotype[82].

Patients with a type L phenotype have preserved pulmonary compliance. This compliance allows these patients to have sufficient minute volumes to maintain blood oxygenation without triggering dyspnoea or respiratory distress. Type H is characterised by high elastance, which is responsible for a picture resembling that of typical ARDS, with severe and early polypnoea, hypoxaemia and bilateral pulmonary infiltrates[83].

On the other hand, polypnoea is predictive of rapid clinical deterioration in relation to the severity of Covid-19 pneumonitis. This same finding was reported by Xie et al[84].

When biological abnormalities were analysed, lymphopenia was found in the majority of our patients (71%). This rate is similar to that found by Guan (83%) and Richardson (60%)[4,65]. This lymphopenia has been explained by the direct cytotoxicity of the virus and the significant release of cytokines inducing cell apoptosis[85].

Although our study did not show an association between lymphopenia and the poor prognosis of patients (p=0.056), this has been found in several studies. In a meta-analysis of 31 studies, lymphopenia was associated with disease severity [86]. These results were comparable to those reported by Tan and Lippi [87,88]. The small size of our population compared with the series reported above may explain the absence of a significant association between lymphopenia and poor prognosis.

The white blood cell count has also been studied in COVID 19 and its prognostic role has been well established [89]. In our study, hyperleukocytosis was present in 27% of cases and was associated with disease progression (p=0.006).

The neutrophil to lymphocyte ratio (NLR) indicates an imbalance in the inflammatory cascade[90]. Its prognostic value has been well established in various conditions such as sepsis, malignant tumours and cardiovascular disease[91-93].

Its prognostic value in SARS-CoV-2 pneumonia has also been reported by several authors. In their work, Ma et al showed that NLR is a factor in the progression to acute respiratory distress syndrome [94]. Liu and Tatum also concluded that this ratio was an independent factor in mortality [95,96]. A more recent study of 12862 patients showed that NLR on admission is a practical and cost-effective parameter for risk stratification of patients and for determining therapeutic management and the efficacy of corticosteroid treatment [97].

In the present study, NLR was an independent factor for poor outcome with an OR equal to 1.8 and a cut-off value equal to 4.9. Similar values were reported by Li et al in a meta-analysis of 13 studies[98]. Thrombocytopenia was present in 12% of our patients. Thrombocytopenia has been explained on the one hand by the direct action of SARS-CoV-2 on bone marrow elements, leading to abnormalities in haematopoiesis, and on the other hand by endothelial lesions triggering the activation and aggregation of platelets in the lung, resulting in high platelet consumption[99]. Other mechanisms have also been suggested by certain authors[100]. Although the percentage of thrombocytopenia in our population was lower than that reported in previous studies, its prognostic value was comparable to that reported in the literature. In a meta-analysis including 1779 patients [99], the risk of a poor outcome was 5 times higher in the presence of thrombocytopenia. In addition to blood count parameters, C-reactive protein (CRP), the inflammation protein par excellence, has been reported to be a poor prognostic factor. R. Smilowitz, in a study of 2782 patients, concluded that there was a strong relationship between CRP and the development of thromboembolic complications, acute renal failure, disease progression and death [101]. Similar results were reported by Danwang et al in a meta-analysis of 31 studies [86]. Consistent with these data, elevated CRP was found in the majority of our patients and was significantly associated with poor outcome (OR=11.3; p<0.0001).In the same spirit, several publications have sought to highlight the role of other markers of inflammation such as IL-6, procalcitonin and ferritin in the prognosis of the disease. These markers were not measured in our patients. With regard to the prognostic value of D-dimer levels, it has been shown that high levels are predictive of severity, mortality and thromboembolic complications in SARS-CoV-2 pneumonia[102-104].

D-dimers reflect the activation of coagulation and fibrinolysis. Coagulation leads to the formation of fibrin clots, while subsequent degradation by the fibrinolytic system generates several degradation products, including D-dimers.

This hypercoagulability has been explained by the inflammatory response triggered by infection with SARS-CoV-2, leading to the overproduction of pro-inflammatory cytokines which are responsible for multi-organ lesions and thrombin production. The main function of thrombin is to form clots by activating platelets and converting fibrinogen into fibrin. During this inflammation, there is also an alteration in the production and hyperconsumption of physiological antithrombotics such as antithrombin m.
This imbalance between the procoagulant and anticoagulant systems predisposes to the development of microthrombi and disseminated intravenous coagulation observed in SARS-CoV-2 pneumonia [105-107]. Indeed, post-mortem analysis of the lungs of 12 patients who died of COVID-19 by Wichmann et al showed a high incidence of deep vein thrombosis, pulmonary embolism and disseminated microthrombi. The development of these in situ thromboses was explained by evidence of impairment of capillary perfusion and direct infection of the endothelium by the virus in association with the inflammatory storm [126].

However, in our study, a high D-dimer level was associated with an unfavourable disease outcome (OR=2.27; p=0.007).

Elevated blood creatinine levels were found in 16.6% of our patients. Similar percentages have been reported in the literature [108]. This impairment of renal function has been described in several studies and has been explained by direct and indirect mechanisms. In fact, SARS-CoV-2 enters human cells via ACE 2, which is present not only on the surface of alveolar cells but also on the surface of renal cells, leading to tubular and glomerular damage. In addition to this direct action, the cytokine storm, Macrophagic activation syndrome and lymphopenia caused by immune dysregulation in COVID19 may be responsible for acute renal failure. Sepsis, rhabdomyolysis and endothelial damage are also potential mechanisms of acute renal failure. Hypoxia can also cause acute renal ischaemia [109]. Malik et al, in a meta-analysis involving 3635 patients, showed that the risk of an unfavourable outcome was 3 times higher in patients with high blood creatinine levels on admission [110]. Similarly, in the study by Bayrakci et al involving 328 patients hospitalised in an intensive care unit, acute renal failure was associated with a high mortality rate (p<0.001) [111]. Our results are in line with those reported in the literature. Liver damage was also observed in patients with SARS-CoV-2 pneumonia, notably in 18.3% of our patients. The pathophysiological mechanisms were comparable to those incriminated in renal disease. However, the pre-existence of chronic liver disease and the use of certain drugs may aggravate this condition [112]. Most recent studies have demonstrated its role in the deterioration of the disease [113,114]. In our study, there was no association between liver damage and poor prognosis. Prognostic studies in SARS-CoV-2 pneumonia have also looked at the impact of rhabdomyolysis on the prognosis of the disease. In a retrospective study of 1014 patients, elevated CPK was significantly associated with clinical deterioration, transfer to intensive care and mortality [115].

In the present study, its incidence was higher (22%) than the figures reported in the literature: 2.2% in the study by Geng et al and only 0.2% in the study by Guan et al, but it had the same prognostic value ($p<0.001$) [65,115].

Just as biological parameters play an important role in predicting poor outcome, radiological parameters remain relevant to study and are of interest both diagnostically and prognostically. Studies have therefore sought to demonstrate the value of thoracic computed tomography for diagnostic purposes. In addition, it offers excellent diagnostic performance, with sensitivity ranging from 60 to 89% and specificity from 24 to 94%. This The variability in specificity between studies has been explained by the stage of the disease, the viral load, the performance of the RT-PCR, in particular the site of the sample, and the reliability of the test [116].

The most characteristic CT lesions in SARS-CoV-2 lung disease are: early-onset ground-glass lesions followed by the appearance of parenchymal condensations, with a generally bilateral, multilobar and peripheral distribution and a predominance in the posterior regions of the lungs. Other anomalies have been reported with a lower prevalence, such as septal thickening, bronchiectasis, crazy paving and the halo sign [117,118]. Our results concur with those of the literature concerning the nature of the lesions and their distribution.

In accordance with our study, the extent of lesions and septal thickening were considered to be two prognostic factors for SARS-CoV-2 pneumonia. On the other hand, Rchid, in his thesis involving 67 patients, showed that lung involvement of more than 35% on the initial scan increased the risk of death and recourse to mechanical ventilation, with an Odds Ratio (OR) of 7.88 [119]. In association with septal thickening, other abnormalities have been reported by Chang and Li as poor prognostic factors such as crazy paving, pericardial effusion and pleural effusion [120,121].

In addition, some authors have focused on the analysis of healthy lung parenchyma rather than affected parenchyma. This analysis has the advantage of taking into account chronic parenchymal abnormalities such as fibrosis and emphysema, and of being correlated with functional residual capacity [122,123].

Thoracic imaging also has an important role to play in screening for thromboembolic complications of COVID pneumonia19. In fact, thoracic angioscan is the gold standard for confirming the diagnosis of pulmonary embolism, which is a frequent complication in this context. Its frequency was 9% in a series including 4244 patients hospitalised in intensive care units for severe SARS-CoV-2 pneumonia and 18% in the series by Poyiadji et al [124,125]. In our study, pulmonary embolism was present in 7.3% of our patients. Nevertheless, 11% of patients were initially put on curative anticoagulation because of the severity of the disease, without being able to confirm or rule out the presence of pulmonary embolism. In addition to pulmonary embolism, cases of unusual arterial thrombosis such as thrombi of the aorta associated with unusual cerebral or peripheral embolisms have been described in the literature.

Two similar cases were observed in our patients. Despite the high incidence of thromboembolic complications in COVID-19, a systematic chest CT scan is not performed as part of the initial work-up. Since the start of the COVID-19 pandemic, more than 13,000 clinical trials have been registered. This research and clinical work has led to a better understanding of the disease and its different phases, and to the evaluation of several therapies. However, an effective direct antiviral treatment is still not available. As a result, early stratification of patients will make it possible to identify those who are most likely to develop unfavourably, and to make a better case for hospitalisation and the type of care required.

In this context, several authors have designed prognostic scales to predict mortality and/or progression to a severe form of the disease. In a systematic review of the literature including 51 studies, Waynants et al studied 66 models, 16 of which were prognostic models. These prognostic models evaluated different populations and appeared to be very heterogeneous, with many potential biases related to the size of the sample. However, a number of elements were systematically included in these stratification scores: Advanced age, associated comorbidities (obesity, diabetes), elevated inflammatory markers (NLR, CRP) and the extent of radiological lesions[126].

In the absence of validated prognostic scores for COVID-19 pneumonia, some healthcare professionals have used prognostic scales validated for acute community-acquired pneumonia, such as the Fine score, the CURB65 score and the SOFA score [127,128]. In Allouche's thesis, which included 170 patients hospitalised at the Charles Nicolle Hospital in Tunis for SARS-CoV-2 pneumonia, a CURB65 score 3 was significantly associated with mortality [129]. Similar results were reported by Rodriguez-Nava et al [130]. In this study, we were able to identify poor prognostic factors for SARS-CoV-2 pneumonia in a multivariate study of a Tunisian population. These factors included clinical parameters such as male sex and high oxygen requirements on admission, and biological parameters such as neutrophil to lymphocyte ratio. A prognostic score taking these 3 factors into account would be an easy and rapid tool that could help us in the initial assessment of severity. and guide us in therapeutic management.

CONCLUSIONS

Since its emergence in December 2019, COVID-19 has caused a global epidemic, with the total number of infected cases exceeding 450 million and mortality estimated at between 2% and 3% according to WHO statistics. It thus constituted a global health problem.

In several countries, particularly Tunisia, the peaks of the epidemic have generated a high demand for hospital beds, mainly in intensive care units. As a result, early identification of clinical and paraclinical parameters predictive of adverse outcomes is of great importance in improving patient care and optimising resource management.

The aim of our work was therefore to study the epidemiological, clinical, biological and radiological characteristics of SARS-CoV-2 pneumonia and to identify factors predictive of an unfavourable outcome.

To this end, we conducted a retrospective, descriptive study including 300 patients admitted to the Pneumology Department B of the Abderrahmane Mami Hospital for management of SARS-CoV-2 pneumonia between October 2020 and April 2021.

The disease was predominantly male, with a sex ratio of 1.38. The median age of our patients was 65 ± 13 years.

Active smoking was common in our patients (44%). The most common comorbidities were arterial hypertension (45.3%), followed by diabetes (39.3%), COPD (15%) and coronary heart disease (12%). Contrary to the literature, none of these comorbidities was associated with a poor prognosis.

Dyspnoea was the main symptom (85.3%) and polypnoea was the most frequent sign on physical examination (50%).

The biological abnormalities noted on the haemogram were lymphopenia (71.3%), hyperleukocytosis (27%), thrombocytopenia (12.3%) and eosinopenia (7.3%). The neutrophil to lymphocyte ratio was greater than 4.9 in 135 patients (45%). Liver cytolysis was found in 47% of patients. Rhabdomyolysis was observed in 23.3% of patients. In terms of renal function, acute renal failure was identified in 41 patients on admission (13.6). D-dimer levels were greater than 500 ng/mL in 65% of cases. Chest CT revealed ground-glass lesions (95.8%), parenchymal condensations (67%) and crazypaving (13.3%). Radiological lesions were extensive in more than half the cases (57.6%).

Oxygen therapy was indicated in all hospitalised patients, with a median flow rate of 6 litres [1-60]. Seventeen per cent of patients had an oxygen requirement15 litres on admission.

The outcome was favourable in 67% of patients, with a mean hospital stay of 9.5 ±6 days, 84 patients were transferred to the intensive care unit (28%) and 16 patients died (6%). The most frequent complication was acute respiratory distress syndrome in 97 patients (32%), followed by acute renal failure in 41 patients (13.6%) and pulmonary embolism in 22 patients (7.3%).

The prognostic factors we identified by univariate analysis were male sex ($p<10^{-3}$), digestive signs($p=0.01$), high oxygen requirements on admission($p<10^{-3}$), higher BMI ($p=0.03$), polypnoea($p<10^{-3}$), parenchymal involvement greater than 50% ($p=0.001$), septal thickening ($p=0.005$) and several biological factors.The biological parameters on admission associated with a poor prognosis were hyperleukocytosis (p=0.006), thrombocytopenia (p=0.013), elevated C-reactive protein (p=0.001), elevated blood creatinine (p=0.007), elevated neutrophil/lymphocyte ratio (p=0.001), elevated d-dimer (p=0.01) and rhabdomyolysis (p<0.001). These data are in line with the literature, which presents these factors as predictive of poor outcome in SARS-CoV-2 pneumonia.The multivariate study looking for independent predictors of poor outcome identified male sex (OR=4.5), oxygen requirements on admission 5.5L/min (OR=2.3) and a neutrophil/lymphocyte ratio 4.9 (OR=1.8) as risk factors. Knowledge of these factors could help clinicians to better define patients who are likely to have an unfavourable prognosis at an early stage of the disease, thus enabling a more targeted and specific approach to preventing poor progression and optimising the management of medical resources. However, the limitations we encountered in carrying out this retrospective study were the lack of certain clinical and/or biological data and the monocentric nature of our study.The prospects for this study would be to extend the sample to a larger scale in order to better determine the prognostic factors of COVID-19 in our population and to establish a prognostic index including these factors. This could help to develop different therapeutic strategies for a more efficient use of the limited medical resources in our country. It is also interesting to carry out post-CoVID follow-up studies to determine the long-term effects of SARS-CoV-2 and its sequelae in patients with COVID-19.

REFERENCES

1. World Health Organization. Coronavirus disease (COVID-19). [On-line]. 2020 [cited 12 April 2022]. Available at: https://www.who.int/fr/health-topics/health- systems-governance

2. World Health Organization. Novel Coronavirus (2019-nCoV) situation reports. [Online]. 2022 [cited 12 April 2022]. Available from: https://www.who.int/fr

3. Hu L, Chen S, Fu Y, Gao Z, Long H, Wang JM, et al. Risk factors associated with clinical outcomes in 323 COVID-19 hospitalized patients in Wuhan, China. Clin Infect Dis. 2020;71(16):2089-98.

4. Richardson S, Hirsch JS, Narasimhan M, Crawford JM, McGinn T, Davidson KW, et al. Presenting characteristics, comorbidities, and outcomes among 5700 patients hospitalized with COVID-19 in the New York city area. J Am Med Assoc. 2020;323(20):2052-9.

5. Garnier M, Quesnel C, Constantin JM. Pulmonary diseases associated with COVID-19. Presse Med. 2021;2(1):14-24.

6. Ministry of Health. Update on the situation in Tunisia. [On-line]. 2020 [cited 12 April 2022]. Available from: http://www.santetunisie.rns.tn/fr/

7. Chen N, Zhou M, Dong X, Qu J, Gong F, Han Y, et al. Epidemiological and clinical characteristics of 99 cases of 2019 novel coronavirus pneumonia in Wuhan, China: a descriptive study. Lancet. 2020;395(10223):507-13.

8. Docherty AB, Harrison EM, Green CA, Hardwick HE, Pius R, Norman L, et al. Features of 20 133 UK patients in hospital with covid-19 using the ISARIC WHO clinical characterisation protocol: prospective observational cohort study. Br Med J. 2020;369:1985.

9. Onder G, Rezza G, Brusaferro S. Case-fatality rate and characteristics of patients dying in relation to COVID-19 in Italy. J Am Med Assoc. 2020;323(18):1775-6.

10. Revel MP, Parkar AP, Prosch H, Silva M, Sverzellati N, Gleeson F, et al. COVID-19 patients and the radiology department - advice from the european society of radiology (ESR) and the european society of thoracic imaging (ESTI). Eur Radiol. 2020;30(9):4903-9.

11. Instance Nationale de l'Evaluation et de l'Accréditation en Santé. Guide parcours du patient suspect ou confirme COVID-19. [On-line]. 2020 [cited 12 April 2022]. Available from: https://www.ineas.tn/

12. Ranieri VM, Rubenfeld G, Thompson B, Ferguson N, Caldwell E, Slutsky AS, et al. Acute respiratory distress syndrome: the berlin definition. J Am Med Assoc. 2012;307(23):2526-33.

13. Jiang S, Shi Z, Shu Y, Song J, Gao GF, Tan W, et al. A distinct name is needed for the new coronavirus. Lancet. 2020;395(10228):949.

14. Louhaichi S, Allouche A, Baili H,Jrad S, Radhouani A,Greb D, et al. Characteristics of patients hospitalised in pneumology for a COVID-19 infection La tunisie Medicale - 2020 ;98 (04) : 261-265.

15. Khadhraoui M. The Covid-19 epidemic in Tunisia in figures [Online]. 2021 [cited

24 March 2022]. Available at: https://inkyfada.com/fr/2021/07/06/covid-19- dashboard-tunisie/.

16. Wu Z, McGoogan JM. Characteristics of and important lessons from the coronavirus disease 2019 (COVID-19) outbreak in china: summary of a report of 72,314 cases from the chinese center for disease control and prevention. J Am Med Assoc. 2020;323(13):1239-42.

17. Zhou F, Yu T, Du R, Fan G, Liu Y, Liu Z, et al. Clinical course and risk factors for mortality of adult inpatients with COVID-19 in Wuhan, China: a retrospective cohort study. Lancet. 2020;395(10229):1054-62.

18. Semenzato L, Botton J, Drouin J, Cuenot F, Weill A, Zureik M. Chronic diseases, health status and risk of hospitalisation and hospital death for COVID-19 during the first wave of the epidemic in France: a cohort study of 66 million people [Online]. 2021 [cited 27 March 2022]. Available from: https://resistance-mondiale.com/wp-content/uploads/2021/10/20210723-report-epiphare-covid-19-hospitalisation-deces.pdf

19. Pan L, Mu M, Yang P, Sun Y, Wang R, Yan J, et al. Clinical characteristics of COVID-19 patients with digestive symptoms in Hubei, China: a descriptive, cross-sectional, multicenter study. Am J Gastroenterol. 2020;115(5):766-73.

20. Jin X, Lian JS, Hu JH, Gao J, Zheng L, Zhang YM, et al. Epidemiological, clinical and virological characteristics of 74 cases of coronavirus-infected disease 2019 (COVID-19) with gastrointestinal symptoms. Gut. 2020;69(6):1002-9.

21. Bienvenu LA, Noonan J, Wang X, Peter K. Higher mortality of COVID-19 in males: sex differences in immune response and cardiovascular comorbidities. Cardiovasc Res. 2020;116(14):2197-206.

22. Mohamed MS, Moulin TC, Schiöth HB. Sex differences in COVID-19: the role of androgens in disease severity and progression. Endocrine. 2021;71(1):3-8.

23. Mjaess G, Karam A, Aoun F, Albisinni S, Roumeguère T. COVID-19 and the male susceptibility: the role of ACE2, TMPRSS2 and the androgen receptor. Prog Urol. 2020;30(10):484-7.

24. Aguilar Pineda JA, Albaghdadi M, Jiang W, Lopez KJV, Del Carpio GD, Valdez BG, et al. Structural and functional analysis of female sex hormones against SARS-Cov2 cell entry. Int J Mol Sci. 2021;22(21):11508.

25. Ding T, Zhang J, Wang T, Cui P, Chen Z, Jiang J, et al. Potential influence of menstrual status and sex hormones on female severe acute respiratory syndrome coronavirus 2 infection:

a cross-sectional multicenter study in Wuhan, China. Clin Infect Dis. 2021;72(9):240-8.

26. Liu D, Ding HL, Chen Y, Chen DH, Yang C, Yang LM, et al. Comparison of the clinical characteristics and mortalities of severe COVID-19 patients between pre- and post-menopause women and age-matched men. Aging. 2021;13(18):21903- 13.

27. Razjouyan J, Helmer DA, Lynch KE, Hanania NA, Klotman PE, Sharafkhaneh A, et al. Smoking Status and Factors associated with COVID-19 In-Hospital Mortality among US Veterans. Nicotine Tob Res. 2022;24(5):785-793.

28. Fakhfakh R, Hsairi M, Maalej M, Achour N. Smoking in Tunisia: behaviour and knowledge. Bull World Health Organ. 2002;80(5):350-6.

30. Zhang JJ, Dong X, Cao YY, Yuan YD, Yang YB, Yan YQ. Clinical characteristics of 140 patients infected with SARS-CoV-2 in Wuhan China. Allergy. 2020;75(7):1730- 41.

31. Simons D, Shahab L, Brown J, Perski O. The association of smoking status with SARS-CoV-2 infection, hospitalisation and mortality from COVID-19: a living rapid evidence review with Bayesian meta-analyses (version 7). Addiction. 2021;116(6):1319-68.

32. Huang C, Wang Y, Li X, Ren L, Zhao J, Hu Y, et al. Clinical features of patients infected with 2019 novel coronavirus in Wuhan, China. Lancet. 2020;395(10223):497-506.

33. Zhang JJ, Dong X, Cao YY, Yuan YD, Yang YB, Yan YQ, et al. Clinical characteristics of 140 patients infected with SARS-CoV-2 in Wuhan, China. Allergy. 2020;75(7):1730-41.

34. Thomas D, Berlin I. Covid-19 and smoking. Arch Mal Coeur Vaiss Pratique. 2021;2021(294):26-9.

35. Farsalinos K, Niaura R, Le Houezec J, Barbouni A, Tsatsakis A, Kouretas D, et al. Editorial: nicotine and SARS-CoV-2: COVID-19 may be a disease of the nicotinic cholinergic system. Toxicol Rep. 2020;7:658-63.

36. Changeux JP, Amoura Z, Rey FA, Miyara M. A nicotinic hypothesis for Covid-19 with preventive and therapeutic implications. C R Biol. 2020;343(1):33-9.

37. Gold MS, Sehayek D, Gabrielli S, Zhang X, McCusker C, Ben Shoshan M. COVID-19 and comorbidities: a systematic review and meta-analysis. Postgrad Med. 2020;132(8):749-55.

38. Yang J, Zheng Y, Gou X, Pu K, Chen Z, Guo Q, et al. Prevalence of comorbidities and its effects in patients infected with SARS-CoV-2: a systematic review and meta- analysis. Int J Infect Dis. 2020;94:91-5.

39. Pranata R, Lim MA, Huang I, Raharjo SB, Lukito AA. Hypertension is associated with increased mortality and severity of disease in COVID-19 pneumonia: a systematic review, meta-analysis and meta-regression. J Renin Angiotensin Aldosterone Syst. 2020;21(2):1470320320926899.

40. Yahia F, Zakhama L, Ben Abdelaziz A. COVID-19 and cardiovascular diseases. Scoping

review study. Tunis Med. 2020;98(4):283-94.

41. Pathangey G, Fadadu PP, Hospodar AR, Abbas AE. Angiotensin-converting enzyme 2 and COVID-19: patients, comorbidities, and therapies. Am J Physiol Lung Cell Mol Physiol. 2021;320(3):301-30.

42. Cinaud A, Sorbets E, Blachier V, Vallee A, Kretz S, Lelong H, et al. Hypertension and COVID-19. Presse Med. 2021;2(1):25-32.

43. Lopes RD, Macedo AS, Moll Bernardes RJ, Feldman A, Arruda GS, De Souza AS, et al. Continuing versus suspending angiotensin-converting enzyme inhibitors and angiotensin receptor blockers: Impact on adverse outcomes in hospitalized patients with severe acute respiratory syndrome coronavirus 2 (SARS-CoV-2)-the BRACE CORONA trial. Am Heart J. 2020;226:49-59.

44. Georges JL, Cochet H, Roger G, Ben Jemaa H, Soltani J, Azowa JB, et al. Association between arterial hypertension, renin angiotensin system inhibitor treatments and severe forms of COVID-19. French prospective single-centre study. Ann Cardiol Angeiol. 2020;69(5):247-54.

45. Hasan SS, Kow CS, Hadi MA, Zaidi SR, Merchant HA. Mortality and disease severity among COVID-19 patients receiving renin-angiotensin system inhibitors: a systematic review and meta-analysis. Am J Cardiovasc Drugs. 2020;20(6):571-90.

46. Kuba K, Imai Y, Rao S, Gao H, Guo F, Guan B, et al. A crucial role of angiotensin converting enzyme 2 (ACE2) in SARS coronavirus-induced lung injury. Nat Med. 2005;11(8):875-9.

47. Mehra MR, Desai SS, Kuy S, Henry TD, Patel AN. Cardiovascular disease, drug therapy, and mortality in Covid-19. N Engl J Med. 2020;382(25):102.

48. Bouhanick B, Cracowski JL, Faillie JL. Diabetes and COVID-19 [Online]. 2020 [cited 12 April 2022]. Available at: https://www.ncbi.nlm.nih.gov/pmc/articles/PMC7194540/

49. Matsushita K, Ding N, Kou M, Hu X, Chen M, Gao Y, et al. The relationship of COVID-19 severity with cardiovascular disease and its traditional risk factors: a systematic review and meta-analysis. Glob Heart. 2020;15(1):64.

50. Fadini GP, Morieri ML, Longato E, Avogaro A. Prevalence and impact of diabetes among people infected with SARS-CoV-2. J Endocrinol Invest. 2020;43(6):867-9.

51. Cariou B, Gourdy P, Hadjadj S, Pichelin M, Wargny M. Diabetes and COVID-19: lessons from CORONADO. Medecine des Maladies Metaboliques. 2021;15(1):15-23.

52. Damayanthi HT, Prabani KP, Weerasekara I. Factors associated for mortality of older people with COVID 19: a systematic review and meta-analysis. Gerontol Geriatr Med. 2021;7:23337214211057392.

53. Alqahtani JS, Oyelade T, Aldhahir AM, Alghamdi SM, Almehmadi M, Alqahtani AS, et

al. Prevalence, severity and mortality associated with COPD and smoking in patients with COVID-19: a rapid systematic review and meta-analysis. PLoS One. 2020;15(5):e0233147.

54. Feng Y, Ling Y, Bai T, Xie Y, Huang J, Li J, et al. COVID-19 with different severities: a multicenter study of clinical features. Am J Respir Crit Care Med. 2020;201(11):1380-8.

55. Javanmardi F, Keshavarzi A, Akbari A, Emami A, Pirbonyeh N. Prevalence of underlying diseases in died cases of COVID-19: a systematic review and meta- analysis. PLoS One. 2020;15(10):e0241265.

56. Leung JM, Niikura M, Yang CT, Sin DD. COVID-19 and COPD. Eur Respir J. 2020;56(2):2002108.

57. Solís P, Carreño H. COVID-19 fatality and comorbidity risk factors among diagnosed patients in Mexico [Online]. 2020 [cited 12 April 2022]. Disponible sur: https://www.medrxiv.org/content/10.1101/2020.04.21.20074591v1

58. Gao Y dong, Ding M, Dong X, Zhang J jin, Kursat Azkur A, Azkur D, et al. Risk factors for severe and critically ill COVID-19 patients: a review. Allergy. 2021;76(2):428-55.

59. Skevaki C, Karsonova A, Karaulov A, Xie M, Renz H. Asthma-associated risk for COVID-19 development. J Allergy Clin Immunol. 2020;146(6):1295-301.

60. Wark PB, Pathinayake PS, Kaiko G, Nichol K, Ali A, Chen L, et al. ACE2 expression is elevated in airway epithelial cells from older and male healthy individuals but reduced in asthma. Respirology. 2021;26(5):442-51.

61. Carr TF, Kraft M. Asthma and atopy in COVID-19: 2021 updates. J Allergy Clin Immunol. 2022;149(2):562-4.

62. Williamson EJ, Walker AJ, Bhaskaran K, Bacon S, Bates C, Morton CE, et al. Factors associated with COVID-19-related death using openSAFELY. Nature. 2020;584(7821):430-6.

63. Hanon S, Brusselle G, Deschampheleire M, Louis R, Michils A, Peché R, et al. COVID-19 and biologics in severe asthma: data from the belgian severe asthma registry. Eur Respir J. 2020;56(6):2002857.

64. Antonicelli L, Tontini C, Manzotti G, Ronchi L, Vaghi A, Bini F, et al. Severe asthma in adults does not significantly affect the outcome of COVID-19 disease: results from the italian severe asthma registry. Allergy. 2021;76(3):902-5.

65. Guan WJ, Ni Z Y, Hu Y, Liang WH, Ou CQ, He JX, et al. Clinical characteristics of coronavirus disease 2019 in China. N Engl J Med. 2020;382(18):1708-20.

66. Plaçais L. COVID-19: clinical, biological and radiological characteristics in adults, pregnant women and children. An update at the heart of the pandemic. Rev Med Interne. 2020;41(5):308-18.

67. Luo S, Zhang X, Xu H. Don't overlook digestive symptoms in patients with 2019 novel

coronavirus disease (COVID-19). Clin Gastroenterol Hepatol. 2020;18(7):1636-7.

68. Hoffmann M, Kleine Weber H, Schroeder S, Krüger N, Herrler T, Erichsen S, et al. SARS-CoV-2 cell entry depends on ACE2 and TMPRSS2 and is blocked by a clinically proven protease inhibitor. Cell. 2020;181(2):271-80.

69. Xiao F, Tang M, Zheng X, Liu Y, Li X, Shan H. Evidence for gastrointestinal infection of SARS-CoV-2. Gastroenterology. 2020;158(6):1831-3.

70. Tian Y, Rong L, Nian W, He Y. Review article: gastrointestinal features in COVID- 19 and the possibility of faecal transmission. Food Pharmacol Ther. 2020;51(9):843-51.

71. Meyiz H, El Jaadi I, Akjay A, Mellouki I. COVID-19 and digestive manifestations: mechanisms and implications during infection. J Med Dent Sci. 2021;20(2):10- 4.

72. Yang J, Hu J, Zhu C. Obesity aggravates COVID-19: a systematic review and meta-analysis. J Med Virol. 2021;93(1):257-61.

73. Lighter J, Phillips M, Hochman S, Sterling S, Johnson D, Francois F, et al. Obesity in patients younger than 60 years is a risk factor for covid-19 hospital admission. Clin Infect Dis. 2020;71(15):896-7.

74. Petrilli CM, Jones SA, Yang J, Rajagopalan H, O'Donnell L, Chernyak Y, et al. Factors associated with hospital admission and critical illness among 5279 people with coronavirus disease 2019 in New York city: prospective cohort study. Br Med J. 2020;369:1966.

75. Simonnet A, Chetboun M, Poissy J, Raverdy V, Noulette J, Duhamel A, et al. High prevalence of obesity in severe acute respiratory syndrome coronavirus-2 (SARS- CoV-2) requiring invasive mechanical ventilation. Obesity. 2020;28(7):1195-9.

76. Chetboun M, Raverdy V, Labreuche J, Simonnet A, Wallet F, Caussy C, et al. BMI and pneumonia outcomes in critically ill COVID-19 patients: an international multicenter study. Obesity. 2021;29(9):1477-86.

77. Czernichow S, Beeker N, Rives Lange C, Guerot E, Diehl J, Katsahian S, et al. Obesity doubles mortality in patients hospitalized for SARS-CoV-2 in Paris hospitals, France: a cohort study on 5795 patients. Obesity. 2020;28(12):2282-9.

78. Caussy C. Obesity and COVID-19 infection: a dangerous link. Medecine des Maladies Metaboliques. 2021;15(3):288-93.

79. Izcovich A, Ragusa MA, Tortosa F, Lavena Marzio MA, Agnoletti C, Bengolea A, et al. Prognostic factors for severity and mortality in patients infected with COVID- 19: a systematic review. PLoS One. 2020;15(11):e0241955.

80. Breville G, Accorroni A, Allali G, Adler D. Pathophysiology of silent hypoxaemia in Covid-19. Rev Med Suisse. 2021;17(736):831-4.

81. Dhont S, Derom E, Van Braeckel E, Depuydt P, Lambrecht BN. The pathophysiology of 'happy' hypoxemia in COVID-19. Respir Res. 2020;21(1):198.

82. Gattinoni L, Camporota L, Marini JJ. COVID-19 phenotypes: leading or misleading? Eur Respir J. 2020;56(2):2002195.

83. Cajanding RM. Silent hypoxia in COVID-19 pneumonia: state of knowledge, pathophysiology, mechanisms, and management. AACN Adv Crit Care. 2022;8(1):1-11.

84. Xie J, Covassin N, Fan Z, Singh P, Gao W, Li G, et al. Association between hypoxemia and mortality in patients with COVID-19. Mayo Clin Proc. 2020;95(6):1138-47.

85. Muller M, Bulubas I, Vogel T. Prognostic factors in Covid-19. NPG Neurology, Psychiatry, Geriatry. 2021;21(125):304-12.

86. Danwang C, Endomba FT, Nkeck JR, Wouna DA, Robert A, Noubiap JJ. A meta-analysis of potential biomarkers associated with severity of coronavirus disease 2019 (COVID-19). Biomark Res. 2020;8:37.

87. Tan L, Wang Q, Zhang D, Ding J, Huang Q, Tang YQ, et al. Lymphopenia predicts disease severity of COVID-19: a descriptive and predictive study. Signal Transduct Target Ther. 2020;5(1):33.

88. Lippi G, Plebani M. The critical role of laboratory medicine during coronavirus disease 2019 (COVID-19) and other viral outbreaks. Clin Chem Lab Med. 2020;58(7):1063-9.

89. Tsoumbou Bakana G, Traore B, Hassoune S, Nani S. Facteurs biologiques predictifs de formes graves de Covid 19 predictive biological factors of severe forms of Covid 19 [On online].2020 [cited12 April 2022]. Available from at: https://revues.imist.ma/index.php/RMSP/article/view/22644

90. Faria SS, Fernandes PC, Silva MB, Lima VC, Fontes W, Freitas Junior R, et al. The neutrophil-to-lymphocyte ratio: a narrative review. Ecancermedicalscience. 2016;10:702.

91. Lagunas Rangel FA. Neutrophil to lymphocyte ratio and lymphocyte to C reactive protein ratio in patients with severe coronavirus disease 2019 (COVID-19): a meta- analysis. J Med Virol. 2020;92(10):1733-4.

92. Meng LB, Yu ZM, Guo P, Wang QQ, Qi RM, Shan MJ, et al. Neutrophils and neutrophil-lymphocyte ratio: inflammatory markers associated with intimal-media thickness of atherosclerosis. Thromb Res. 2018;170:45-52.

93. Huang Z, Fu Z, Huang W, Huang K. Prognostic value of neutrophil-to-lymphocyte ratio in sepsis: a meta-analysis. Am J Emerg Med. 2020;38(3):641-7.

94. Ma A, Cheng J, Yang J, Dong M, Liao X, Kang Y. Neutrophil to lymphocyte ratio as a predictive biomarker for moderate severe ARDS in severe COVID-19 patients. Crit Care. 2020;24(1):288.

95. Tatum D, Taghavi S, Houghton A, Stover J, Toraih E, Duchesne J. Neutrophil-to-lymphocyte ratio and outcomes in Louisiana COVID-19 patients. Shock. 2020;54(5):652-8.

96. Liu Y, Du X, Chen J, Jin Y, Peng L, Wang HX, et al. Neutrophil-to-lymphocyte ratio as an independent risk factor for mortality in hospitalized patients with COVID-19. J Infect. 2020;81(1):6-12.

97. Cai J, Li H, Zhang C, Chen Z, Liu H, Lei F, et al. The neutrophil-to-lymphocyte ratio determines clinical efficacy of corticosteroid therapy in patients with COVID-19. Cell Metab. 2021;33(2):258-69.

98. Li X, Liu C, Mao Z, Xiao M, Wang L, Qi S, et al. Predictive values of neutrophil-to-lymphocyte ratio on disease severity and mortality in COVID-19 patients: a systematic review and meta-analysis. Crit Care. 2020;24(1):647.

99. Lippi G, Plebani M, Henry BM. Thrombocytopenia is associated with severe coronavirus disease 2019 (COVID-19) infections: a meta-analysis. Clin Chim Acta. 2020;506:145-8.

100.Mei H, Luo L, Hu Y. Thrombocytopenia and thrombosis in hospitalized patients with COVID-19. J Hematol Oncol. 2020;13(1):161.

101. Smilowitz NR, Kunichoff D, Garshick M, Shah B, Pillinger M, Hochman JS, et al. C-reactive protein and clinical outcomes in patients with COVID-19. Eur Heart J. 2021;42(23):2270-9.

102.Lippi G, Favaloro EJ. D-dimer is associated with severity of coronavirus disease 2019: a pooled analysis. Thromb Haemost. 2020;120(5):876-8.

103.Bi X, SU Z, Yan H, Du J, Wang J, Chen L, et al. Prediction of severe illness due to COVID-19 based on an analysis of initial fibrinogen to albumin ratio and platelet count. Platelets. 2020;31(5):674-9.

104.Korkusuz R, Karandere F, Senoglu S, Kocoglu H, Yasar KK. The prognostic role of D-dimer in hospitalized COVID-19 patients. Bratisl Lek Listy. 2021;122(11):811-5.

105.Kwaan HC, Mazar AP. More on the source of D-dimer in COVID-19. Thromb Haemost. 2022;122(1):158-9.

106.Zineb EL. Meta-analysis of COVID 19 disease: risk factors and prognostic value of D-dimer [Dissertation]. Medicine: Rabat: 2019. 62p.

107.Bikdeli B, Madhavan MV, Jimenez D, Chuich T, Dreyfus I, Driggin E, et al. COVID-19 and thrombotic or thromboembolic disease: implications for prevention, antithrombotic therapy, and follow-up. J Am Coll Cardiol. 2020;75(23):2950-73.

108.Gtowacka M, Lipka S, Mtynarska E, Franczyk B, Rysz J. Acute kidney injury in COVID-19. Int J Mol Sci. 2021;22(15):8081.

109.Ahmadian E, Hosseiniyan Khatibi SM, Razi Soofiyani S, Abediazar S, Shoja MM, Ardalan M, et al. Covid-19 and kidney injury: pathophysiology and molecular mechanisms. Rev Med Virol. 2021;31(3):e2176.

110.Malik P, Patel U, Mehta D, Patel N, Kelkar R, Akrmah M, et al. Biomarkers and outcomes of COVID-19 hospitalisations: systematic review and meta-analysis. BMJ Evid Based Med. 2021;26(3):107-8.

111.Bayrakci N, Özkan G, akaci M, Sedef S, Erdem i, Tuna N, et al. The incidence of acute kidney injury and its association with mortality in patients diagnosed with COVID-19 followed up in intensive care unit [Online]. 2021 [cited 12 April 2022]. Available Available from: https://www.researchgate.net/profile/Nergiz-Bayrakci/publication/357643595_The_incidence_of_acute_kidney_injury_and_its_association_with_mortality_in_patients_diagnosed_with_COVID_-19_followed-up_in_intensive_care_unit/links/61ea5b7f5779d35951c248d7/The-incidence-of-acute-kidney-injury-and-its-association-with-mortality-in-patients-diagnosed-with-COVID-19-followed-up-in-intensive-care-unit.pdf

112.Nardo AD, Schneeweiss Gleixner M, Bakail M, Dixon ED, Lax SF, Trauner M. Pathophysiological mechanisms of liver injury in COVID-19. Liver Int. 2021;41(1):20-32.

113.Metawea MI, Yousif WI, Moheb I. COVID 19 and liver: an A-Z literature review. Dig Liver Dis. 2021;53(2):146-52.

114.Ding ZY, Li GX, Chen L, Shu C, Song J, Wang W, et al. Association of liver abnormalities with in-hospital mortality in patients with COVID-19. J Hepatol. 2021;74(6):1295-302.

115.Geng Y, Ma Q, Du YS, Peng N, Yang T, Zhang SY, et al. Rhabdomyolysis is associated with in-hospital mortality in patients with COVID-19. Shock. 2021;56(3):360-7.

116.Pontone G, Scafuri S, Mancini ME, Agalbato C, Guglielmo M, Baggiano A, et al. Role of computed tomography in COVID-19. J Cardiovasc Comput Tomogr. 2021;15(1):27-36.

117.Zhou X, Pu Y, Zhang D, Xia Y, Guan Y, Liu S, et al. CT findings and dynamic imaging changes of COVID-19 in 2908 patients: a systematic review and meta-analysis. Acta Radiol. 2022;63(3):291-310.

118.Fields BK, Demirjian NL, Dadgar H, Gholamrezanezhad A. Imaging of COVID-19: CT, MRI, and PET. Semin Nucl Med. 2021;51(4):312-20.

119.Rchid LM. Prognostic value of thoracic computed tomography in patients hospitalized for COVID 19 pneumopathy [Thesis]. Medicine: Marseille; 2020. 55p.

120.Chang MC, Park YK, Kim BO, Park D. Risk factors for disease progression in COVID-19 patients. BMC Infect Dis. 2020;20(1):445.

121.Li K, Wu J, Wu F, Guo D, Chen L, Fang Z, et al. The clinical and chest CT features associated with severe and critical COVID-19 pneumonia. Invest Radiol. 2020;55(6):327-31.

122.Colombi D, Bodini FC, Petrini M, Maffi G, Morelli N, Milanese G, et al. Well-aerated lung on admitting chest CT to predict adverse outcome in COVID-19 pneumonia. Radiology. 2020;296(2):86-96.

123.Nishiyama A, Kawata N, Yokota H, Sugiura T, Matsumura Y, Higashide T, et al. A predictive factor for patients with acute respiratory distress syndrome: CT lung volumetry of the well-aerated region as an automated method. Eur J Radiol. 2020;122:108748.

124.COVID-ICU Group on behalf of the REVA Network and the COVID-ICU Investigators. Clinical characteristics and day-90 outcomes of 4244 critically ill adults with COVID-19: a prospective cohort study. Intensive Care Med. 2021;47(1):60-73.

125.Poyiadji N, Cormier P, Patel PY, Hadied MO, Bhargava P, Khanna K, et al. Acute pulmonary embolism and COVID-19. Radiology. 2020;297(3):335-8.

126.Wynants L, Van Calster B, Collins GS, Riley RD, Heinze G, Schuit E, et al. Prediction models for diagnosis and prognosis of covid-19: systematic review and critical appraisal. Br Med J. 2020;369:1328.

127.Fan G, Tu C, Zhou F, Liu Z, Wang Y, Song B, et al. Comparison of severity scores for COVID-19 patients with pneumonia: a retrospective study. Eur Respir J. 2020;56(3):2002113.

128.Satici C, Demirkol MA, Sargin Altunok E, Gursoy B, Alkan M, Kamat S, et al. Performance of pneumonia severity index and CURB-65 in predicting 30-day mortality in patients with COVID-19. Int J Infect Dis. 2020;98:84-9.

129.Allouche A. SARS-CoV-2 pneumonia. Factors predictive of severity [Thesis]. Medicine: Tunis; 2022. 60p.].

130.RodriguezNava G, Yanez Bello MA, TrellesGarcia DP, Chung CW, Friedman HJ, Hines DW. Performance of the quick COVID-19 severity index and the bresciaCOVID respiratory severity scale in hospitalized patients with COVID-19 in a community hospital setting. Int J Infect Dis. 2021;102:571-6.

APPENDICES

Appendix 1: Body mass index

BMI (kg/ m2)	Interpretation
Less than 18.5	Leanness
18,5 à 25	Normal weight
25 à 30	Overweight
30 à 35	Moderate obesity
35 à 40	Severe obesity
40 and over	Morbid obesity

Appendix 2: Clinical forms of SARS-CoV-2 pneumonia

Forme clinique	Définition	Conduite
Forme asymptomatique	RT-PCR positive sans signes cliniques	Pas d'hospitalisation
Forme mineure	Pas de pneumonie, Toux sèche légère, malaise, céphalées, douleurs musculaires, anosmie, agueusie, pas de dyspnée	Pas d'hospitalisation
Forme modérée	Pneumonie sans signe de sévérité (toux, dyspnée légère, FR < 30 cpm, SpO2 ≥ 94%)	Surveillance rapprochée Hospitalisation en médecine si co-morbidité
Forme sévère	Dyspnée, FR ≥ 30 cpm et/ou SpO2 < 94% à l'air ambiant	Hospitalisation
Forme critique	Détresse vitale, choc, sepsis et/ou défaillance d'organe et/ou la nécessité d'une assistance respiratoire invasive ou non invasive	Hospitalisation en réanimation

Appendix 3: Acute respiratory distress syndrome: Berlin criteria

SDRA : définition de Berlin

Syndrome de détresse respiratoire aiguë
Délai de survenue 1 semaine après une agression pulmonaire ou une aggravation respiratoire
Imagerie thoracique (radiographie ou scanner) Opacités bilatérales non expliquées en totalité par des épanchements, atélectasies ou nodules
Origine de l'œdème Défaillance respiratoire pas totalement expliquée par une défaillance cardiaque ou un excès de remplissage (si pas de facteur de risque de SDRA, évaluation objective de la fonction cardiaque ex : échocardiographie)
Oxygénation **SDRA léger** 200 mmHg < $PaO_2/FiO_2 \leq$ 300 mmHg avec PEEP ou CPAP ≥ 5 cmH_2O
SDRA modéré 100 mmHg < $PaO_2/FiO_2 \leq$ 200 mmHg avec PEEP ≥ 5 cmH_2O
SDRA sévère $PaO_2/FiO_2 \leq$ 100 mmHg avec PEEP ≥ 5 cmH_2O

PEEP : positive end-expiratory pressure
CPAP : continuous positive airway pressure

Appendix 4: Typical CT images of COVID-19 pneumonitis

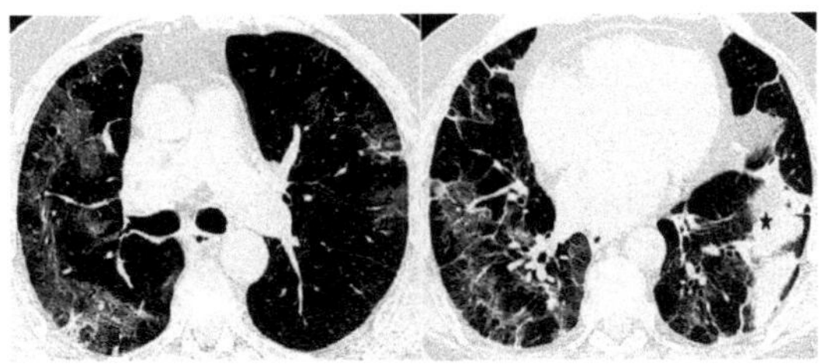

Axial sections of two chest scans showing ground-glass images (arrow), condensations (star) and crazy-paving (arrowheads).

Appendix 5: Different degrees of involvement in COVID-19 pneumopathy

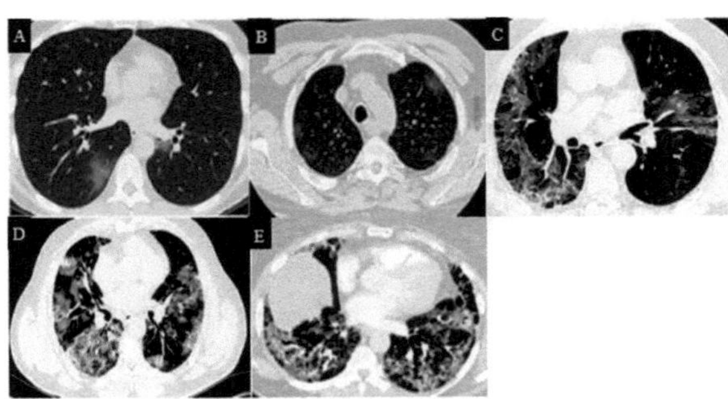

Pulmonary involvement is classified as minimal <10% (A), moderate 10-25% (B), significant 25-50% (C), severe 50-75% (D) and critical >75% (E).

Appendix 6: Complications associated with SARS-CoV-2 pneumonia as seen on thoracic CT scan

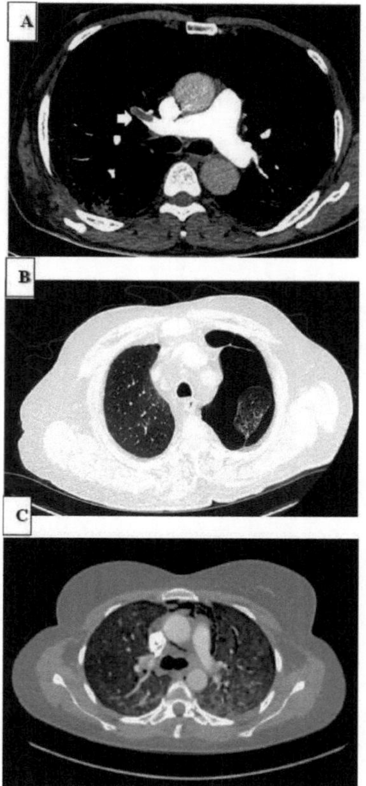

COVID19 pneumonia associated with proximal right pulmonary embolism (A), pneumothorax (B), pneumomediastinum (C).

Appendix 7: Illustration of the mechanisms of coagulopathy in COVID19

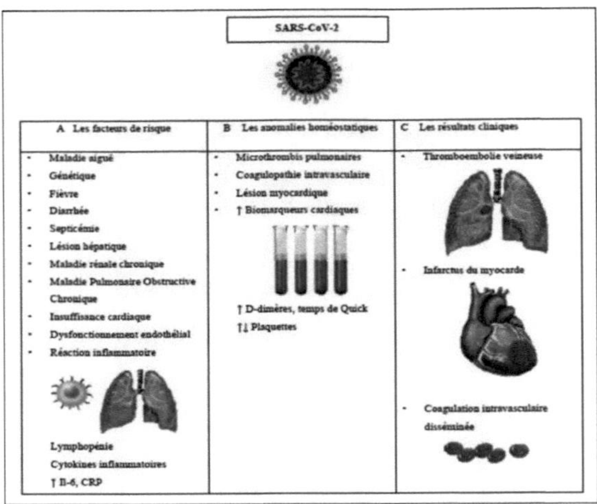

SARS-COV-2 PNEUMONIA IN THE PULMONARY DEPARTMENT: PREDICTIVE FACTORS OF DISEASE PROGRESSION

ABSTRACT

Introduction:

SARS-CoV-2 pneumonia is a serious emerging disease. More than 6 million deaths have been reported by the World Health Organization since the beginning of the pandemic. Identification of factors associated with disease exacerbation is necessary to improve medical resource utilization and to reduce mortality. The aim of our study was to evaluate the epidemiological, clinical, biological, and radiological characteristics of SARS-CoV-2 pneumonia in patients hospitalized in a pulmonary department and to identify predictive factors of an unfavorable short-term evolution.

Methods:

A retrospective and descriptive study including patients hospitalized at the Pneumology Department B of Abderrahmane Mami Hospital for confirmed SARS-CoV-2 pneumonia between October 2020 and April 2021.

Results:

We included 300 patients with a median age of 65±13 years. The sex ratio was 1.38. Male gender was associated with worsening of the disease ($p < 10^{-3}$). The most frequent comorbidities were: arterial hypertension (45.3%), diabetes (39.9%), chronic obstructive pulmonary disease (15%) and coronary artery disease (12%). High oxygen requirements on admission were associated with poor outcome ($p < 10^{-3}$). Biological disorder on admission related to clinical deterioration were hyperleukocytosis (p=0.006), thrombocytopenia (p=0.013), elevated C-reactive protein ($p < 10^{-3}$). ³), elevated neutrophil to lymphocyte ratio (p=0.001), elevated D-dimer (p=0.01), elevated blood creatinine (p=0.007), and rhabdomyolysis ($p < 10^{-3}$). In multivariate analysis, the independent prognostic factors identified were: Male gender (OR=4.5; 95% CI:2.04-10.1; p=0.001), admission oxygen requirements 5.5 L/min (OR=2.3; 95% CI:2.1-3.4; $p<10^{-3}$) and neutrophil/lymphocyte ratio4.9 (OR=1.8; 95% CI:1.09-3.04; p=0.01).

Conclusion:

Male gender, admission oxygen requirement 5.5 L/min and neutrophil/lymphocyte ratio 4.9 are associated with a more guarded prognosis of SARS-CoV-2 pneumonia. The identification of these risk factors, which can be easily used in clinical practice, could help clinicians identify patients with SARS-CoV-2 pneumonia. with poor prognosis at an early stage and optimize the management of medical resources.

Key words: Viral pneumonia, SARS-CoV-2, Severity, Risk factor, Prognosis

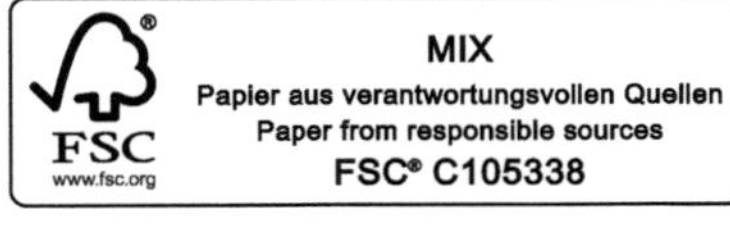

Printed by Books on Demand GmbH, Norderstedt / Germany